Puree Recipes That Loaded with Flavor

Puree Recipes for The Whole Family

BY: Ivy Hope

Copyright © 2020 by Ivy Hope

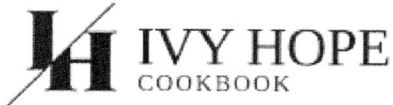

Copyright/License Page

Please don't reproduce this book. It means you are not allowed to make any type of copy (print or electronic), sell, publish, disseminate or distribute. Only people who have written permission from the author are allowed to do so.

This book is written by the author taking all precautions that the content is true and helpful. However, the reader needs to be careful about his/her action. If anything happens due to the reader's actions the author won't be taken as responsible.

Table of Contents

Introduction 5

    Super Green Puree 6

    Orange puree 8

    Purple puree 10

    Carrot Purée 12

    Cauliflower Puree 14

    Sweet Potato Puree 16

    Parsnip Purée 18

    Roasted Butternut Squash Puree 20

    Winter Root Vegetable Puree 22

    First Baby Peas 24

    Papaya 26

    Creamy Provencal Chicken 28

    Carrot, Mango, and Apple Puree 30

    Chayote 32

    Cream of Mushroom Puree 34

Beef Stew for Babies 36

Sugar- free Fig Puree 38

Potato Puree with Garlic 40

Lamb Puree 42

Really Easy Apple Puree 44

Watermelon 46

Zucchini Baby Food Puree 48

White Bean Puree 50

Peach Puree 52

Tomato Puree Recipe 54

Chicken, Rice, and Carrot 56

Strawberry Puree 58

Cooked Strawberry Puree 60

Cherry Puree 62

Plum Puree 64

Conclusion 66

About the Author 67

Author's Afterthoughts 68

Introduction

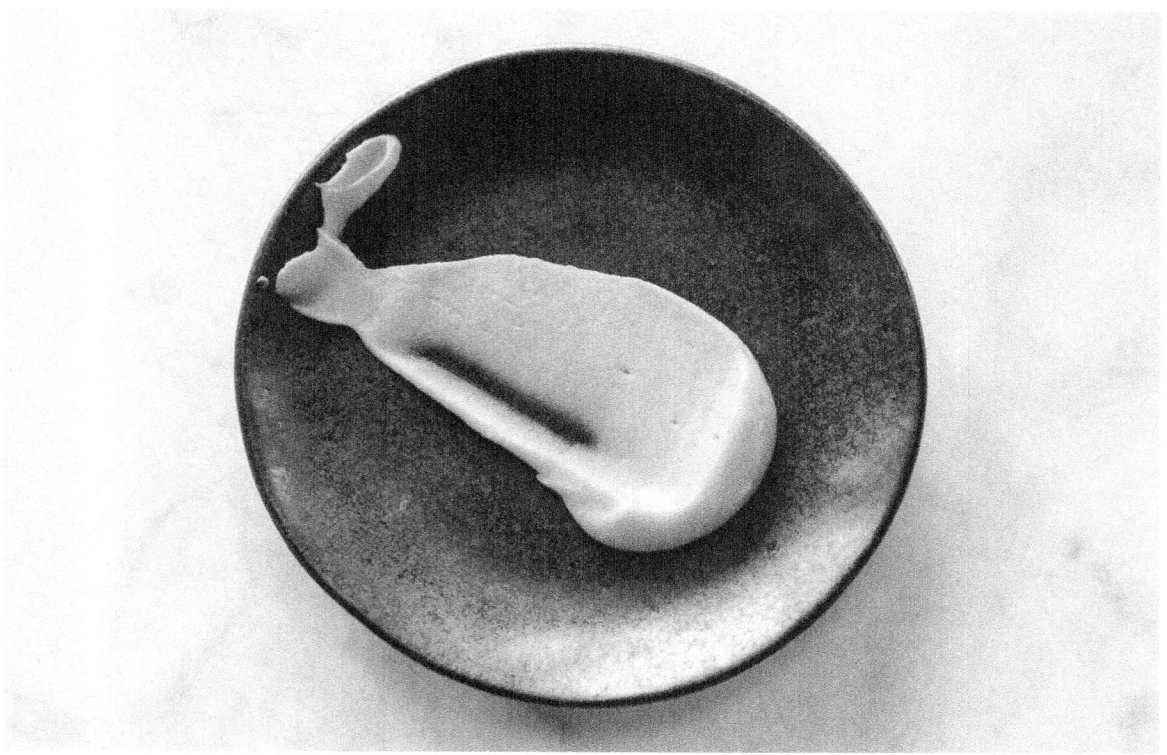

These recipes are fast and simple, featuring herbs, vegetables, fruits, and more flavors. There are 30 awesome recipes in this book for purees. This means everyone will have a favorite puree in no time.

Super Green Puree

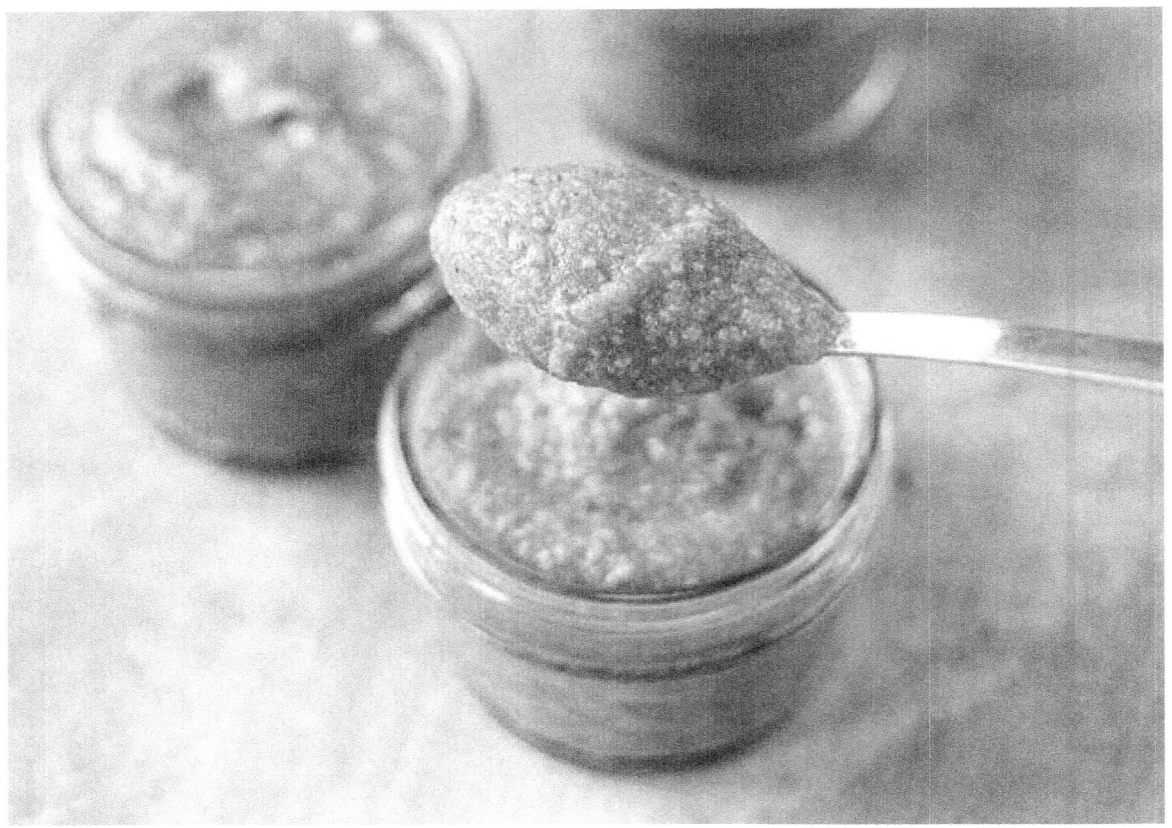

This is a cream and thick puree. It can be severed as a side dish or a dip for crackers. If making has a dip, use less water.

Ingredients

- 2 cups broccoli florets, fresh
- 2 cups raw baby spinach, well rinsed
- 1 cup frozen sweet green peas
- 3 tablespoons water

Directions

Steam broccoli until soft.

Add the peas for two minutes.

Then drain both of them.

In the blender add water, spinach, peas and broccoli blend on high for 2 minutes or until smooth.

Orange puree

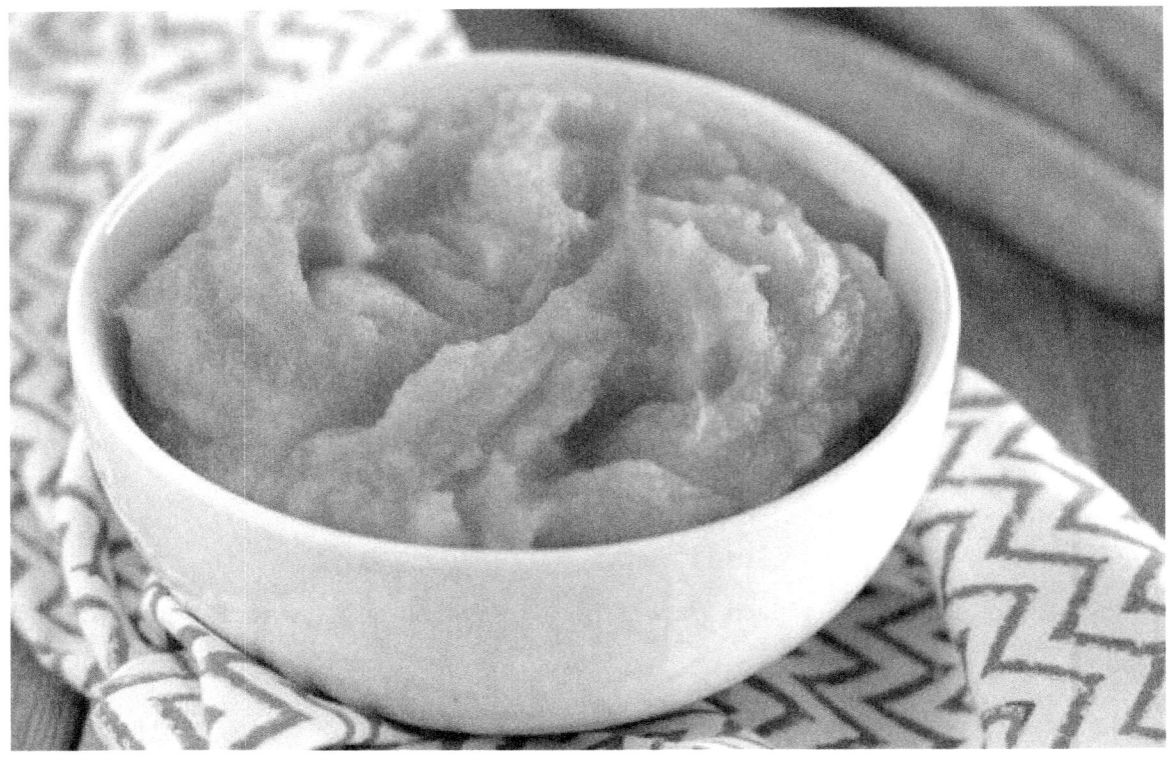

This fruit puree is made 100% fresh organic sweet potatoes and carrots. It's very bright in orange color.

Ingredients

- 1 medium organic sweet potato, peeled and chopped
- 3 large organic carrots, peeled and sliced into thick chunks
- 2 cups of water

Directions

Boil the sweet potato and carrots in 2 cups of water until.

Then drain off the water.

In a food processor, place the sweet potato and carrots.

Puree on high for 1 minute or until smooth.

Water can add a tablespoon at a time to smooth the puree.

Purple puree

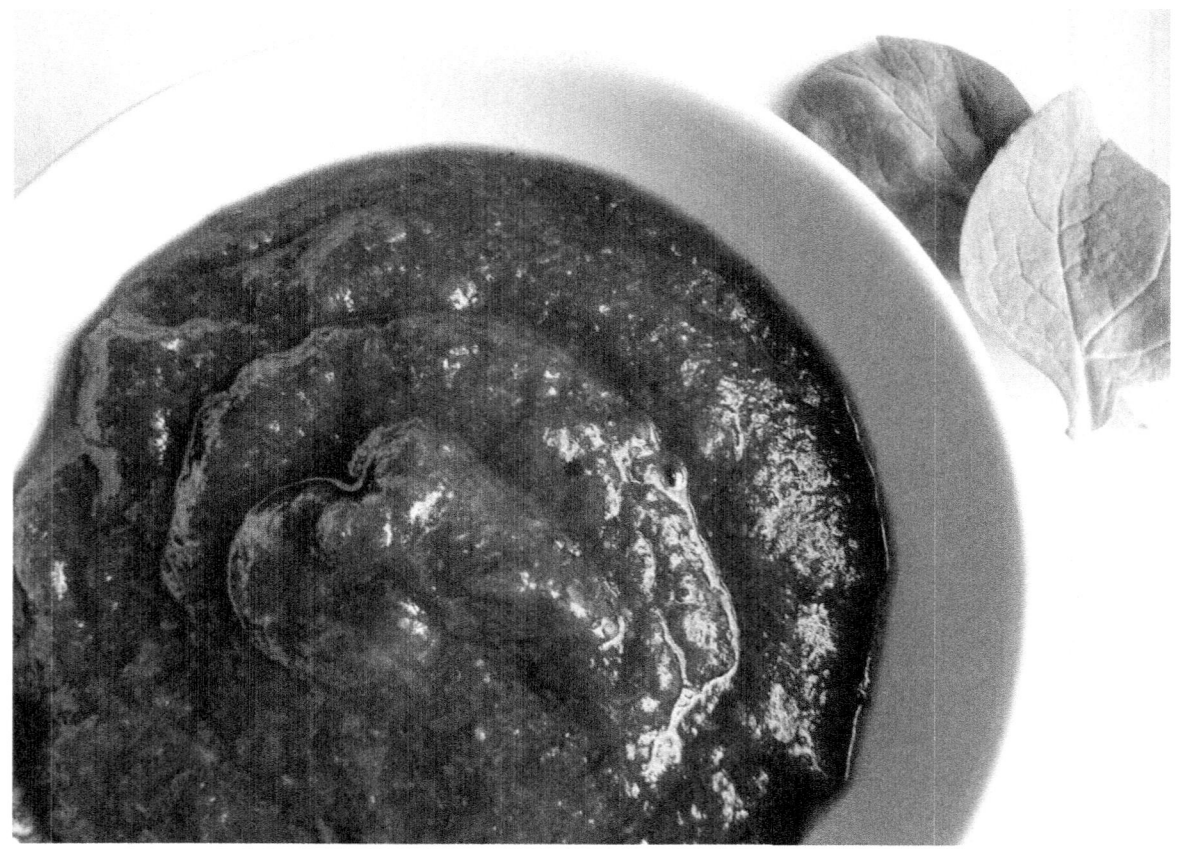

The blueberries give this puree a fun purple color. The best part is the kids will eat it and never know it has vegetables.

Ingredients

- 3 cups organic raw baby spinach
- 1 1/2 cups fresh blueberries, no sugar
- 1/2 teaspoon lemon juice
- 2 tablespoons of tap water

Directions

Rinse the blueberries under cold water.

Place the blueberries to the side to drain.

In the blender add the spinach and blend for 20 seconds on high.

Add the lemon juice, blueberries, and 1 tablespoon water.

Blend on high until smooth and thick.

Carrot Purée

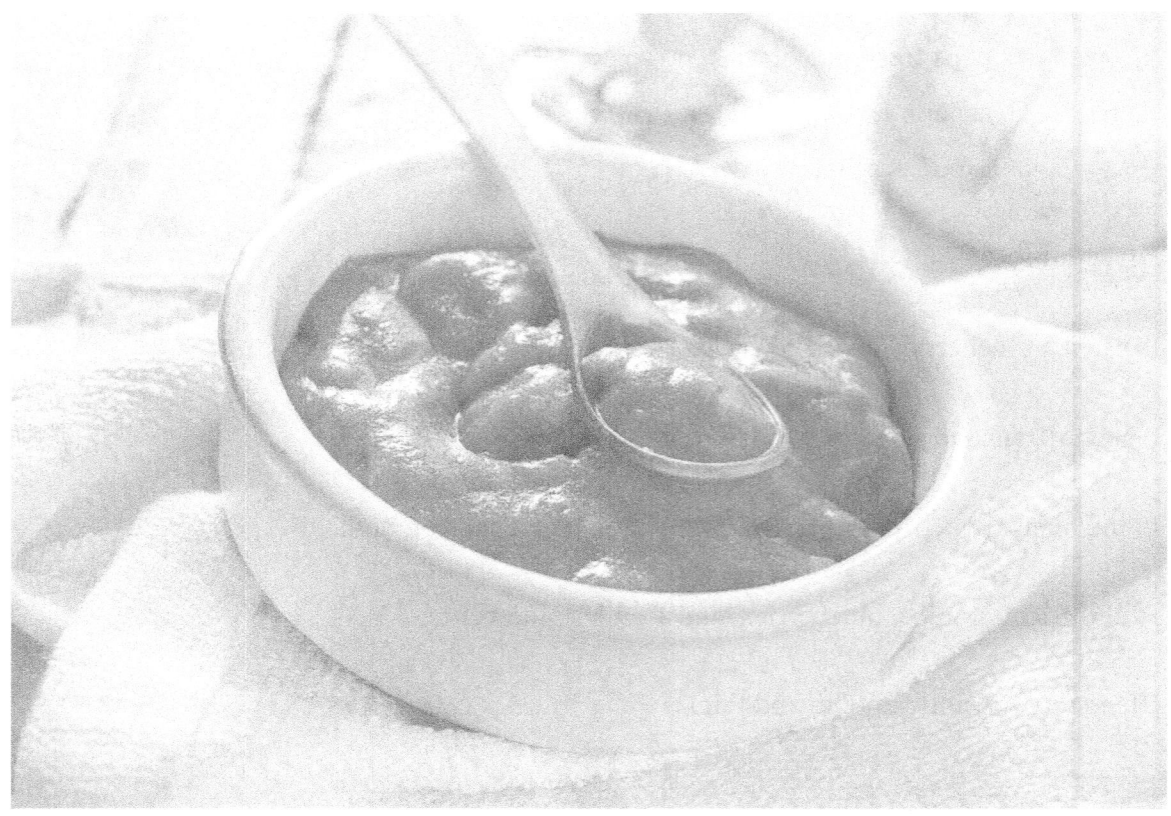

Carrot puree is really good on a fall day served warm. You can pour it into a cup and eat it with some toast.

Ingredients

- 2 cups peeled sliced carrots
- 1 cup chicken broth
- 3 cup clarified butter
- 1 tablespoon chopped chives
- Salt to taste
- Pepper to taste

Directions

Put a small pot on the cooktop and turn the flame to high heat.

Combine the broth and carrots, bring to a boil.

Once boiling drop the heat and simmer with a lid on the pot.

Cook for 8 minutes or until carrots is tender.

Remove the pot from the heat and pour into a bowl.

In the bowl add the butter and mix until smooth using a hand mixer.

Add the salt, pepper, and chives, stir with a spoon until combined.

Cauliflower Puree

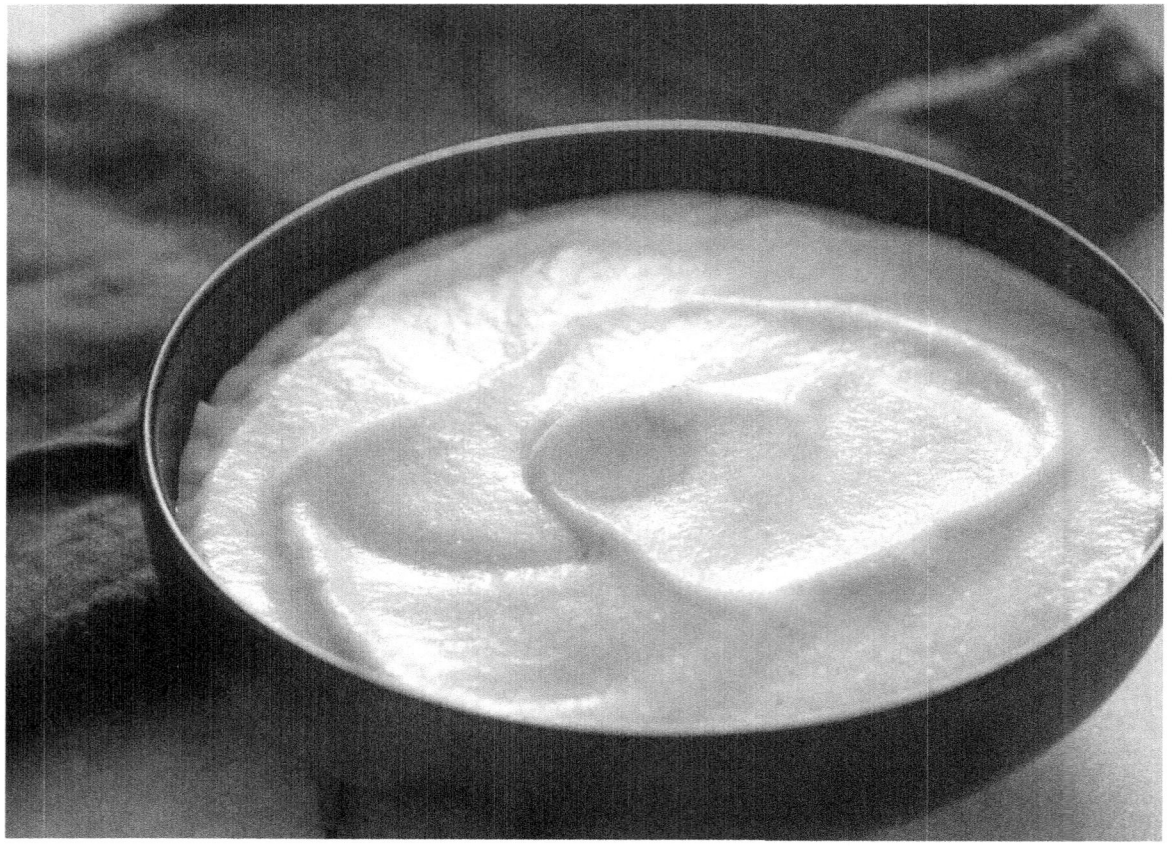

This cauliflower recipe is packed full of flavor. Cauliflower is no longer boiled.

Ingredients

- 5 cups cauliflower leaves and core removed, cut into small florets
- 6 Tablespoons ghee, room temp
- 1/3 Cup chicken stock heated
- 1 teaspoon Sea salt
- 1 teaspoon freshly ground pepper
- 1 teaspoon thyme, chopped

Directions

In a vegetable, steamer and add 2 inches of tap water and add cauliflower.

Place the steamer on the stove and turn the burner to high setting.

Allow the cauliflower to steam until fork tender. Should take no more than 12 minutes. Cool for 5 minutes

Heat the broth in the microwave for 2 minutes and add the ghee and stir.

Once combined pour into a food processor and add the cauliflower.

Puree until smooth and creamy.

Sweet Potato Puree

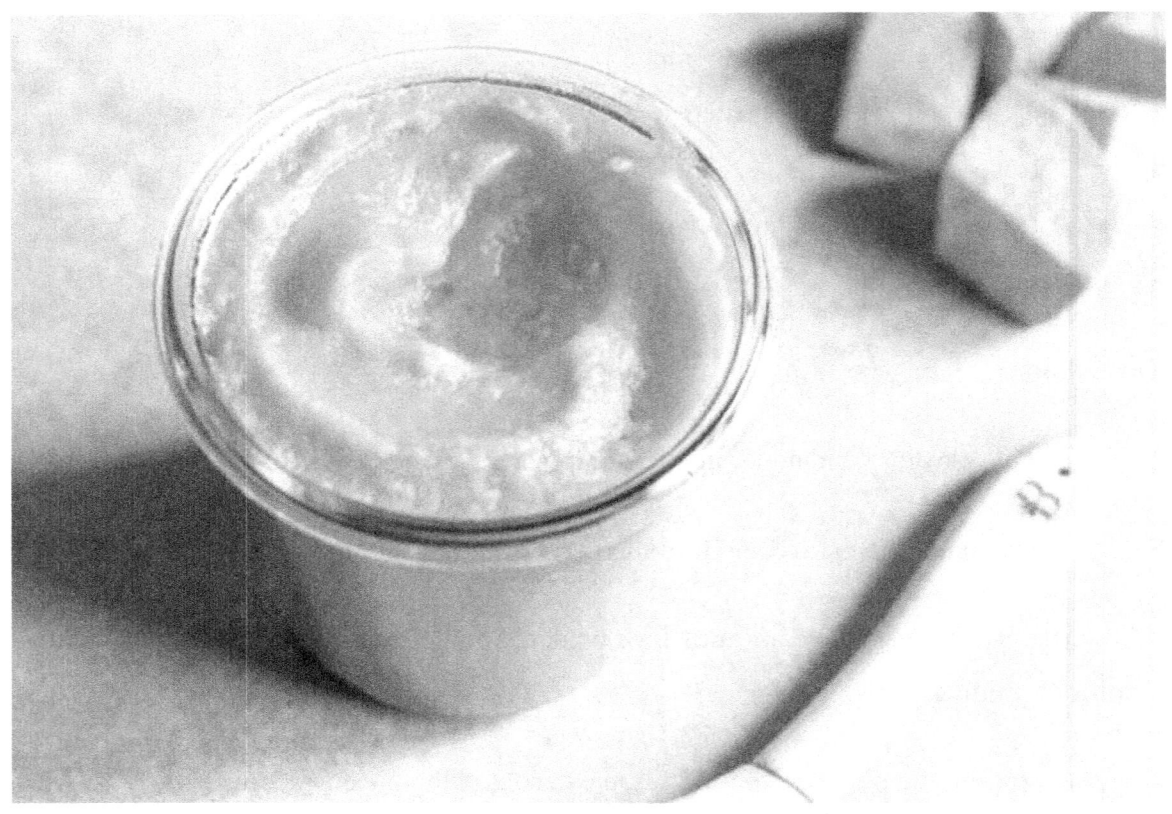

This recipe brings out the creamy taste of Sweet potatoes.

Ingredients

- 4 large fresh sweet potatoes peeled and cubed
- 1/3 cup butter
- 1/3 cup chicken broth
- 1 teaspoon salt
- Pepper to taste

Directions

Set a large pot of water on a high flame.

Bring water to a rapid boil and add the sweet potatoes.

Continue to boil for fork tender.

Remove from heat and dry the water from potatoes. Be careful not to get burnt by the steam.

In a blender, cup add the sweet potatoes, broth, butter, salt, and pepper.

Blend on puree setting until smooth and creamy.

Parsnip Purée

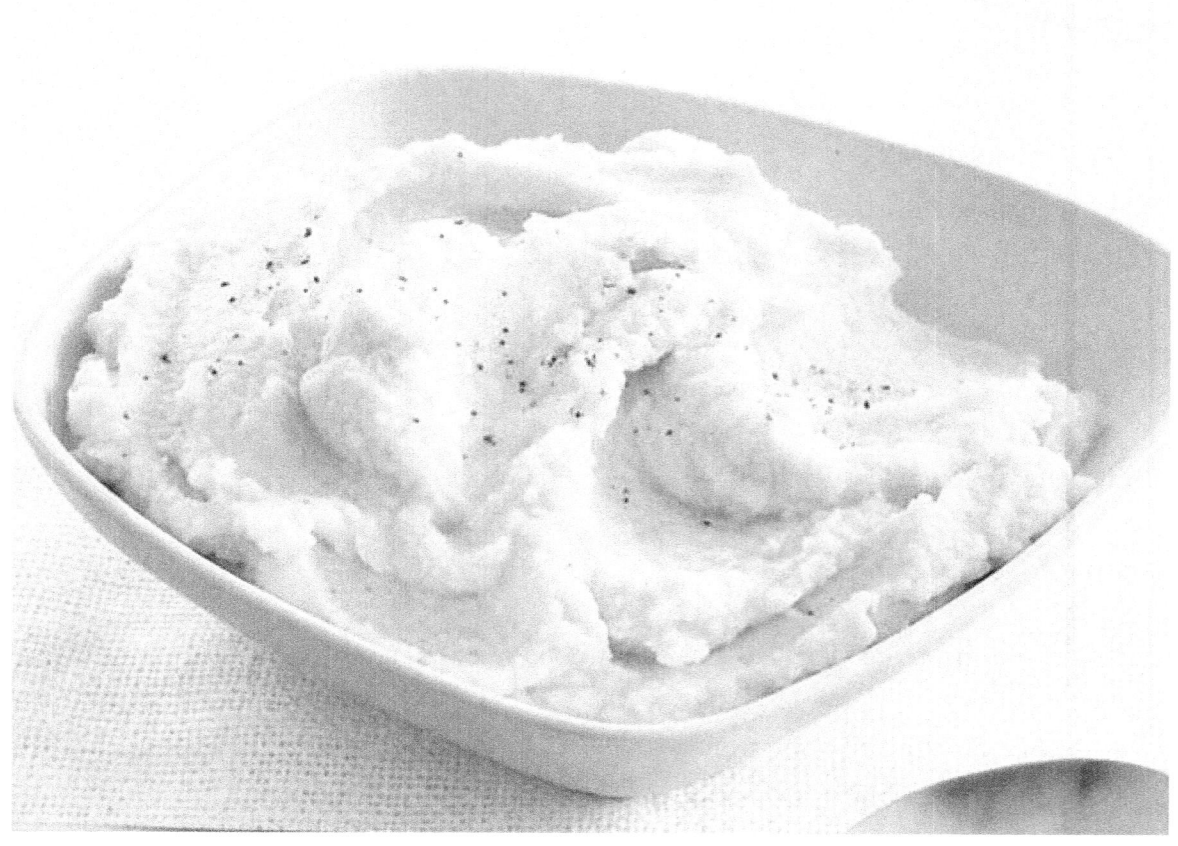

One way to eat the one of delicious puree.

Ingredients

- 2 cups parsnips, peeled sliced (about 1/4 inch thick)
- 1 cup chicken broth
- 1/3 cup clarified butter (use whole 30 use clarified butter)

Directions

Put a small pot on stove burner set on high heat.

Add the broth and parsnips.

Bring broth and parsnips to a boil, then lower the heat to a simmer.

Cook without a lid for 8 minutes. The broth will dissolve. There is no need to worry.

Once parsnips have cooked remove from heat.

Empty into a food processor along with the butter pulse until smooth.

Add salt and pepper, then pour into a bowl and sever.

Roasted Butternut Squash Puree

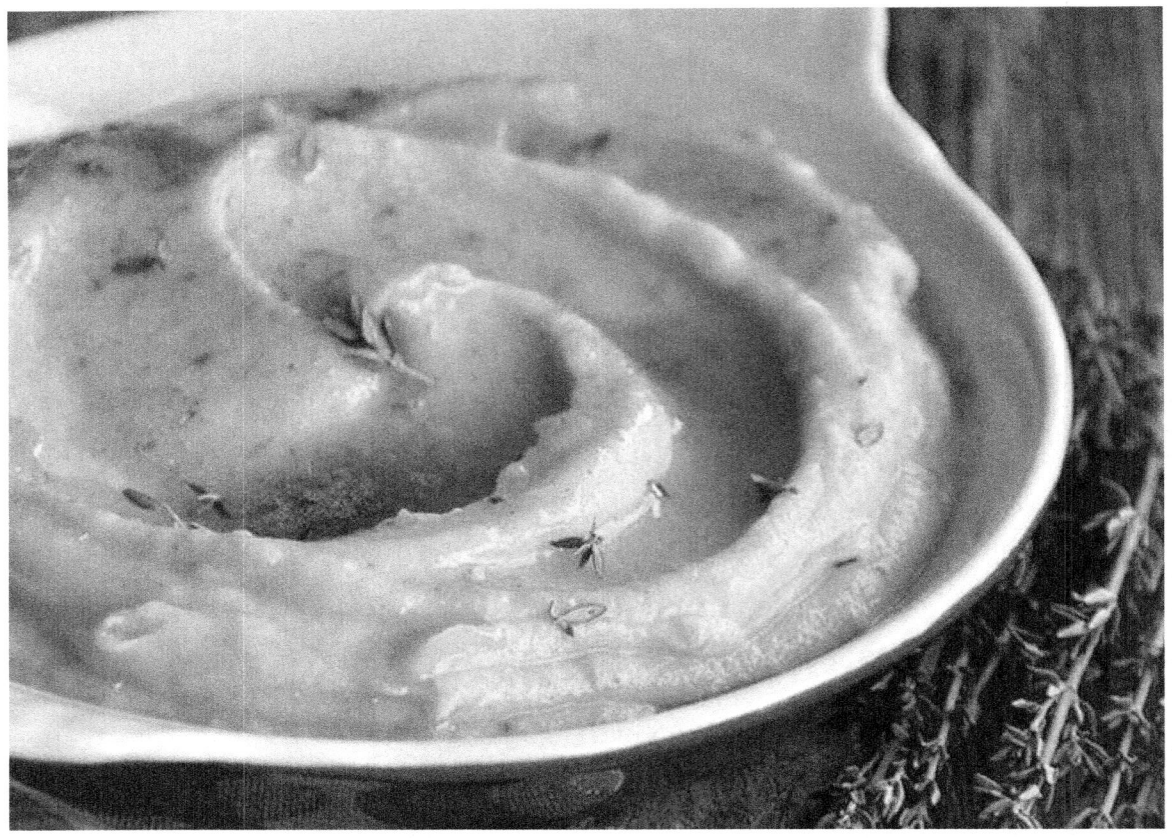

This recipe is always great for a Thanksgiving side dish.

Ingredients

- 3 cups butternut squash peeled and cubed
- 1/2 cup chicken stock
- 1 tablespoon ghee butter
- 2 tablespoon olive oil
- 1 teaspoon salt
- 1 teaspoon freshly ground pepper

Directions

Preheat the oven to 400f and put the oven rack in the upper third slot in oven.

Line a cookie sheet with a parchment paper and place to the side.

Peel the butternut squash, dip out the seeds, in half and cut into ½ inch cubes.

Put the squash onto the parchment covered cookie sheet.

Cover the squash with the oil, salt and pepper.

Place into the oven and roast for 40-45 minutes.

Remove the cookie sheet from the oven and cool for 5 minutes.

Pour squash into a blender add the ghee butter, chicken stock, pepper and salt blend on medium or 2 minutes or until smooth.

Pour into a bowl and serve.

Winter Root Vegetable Puree

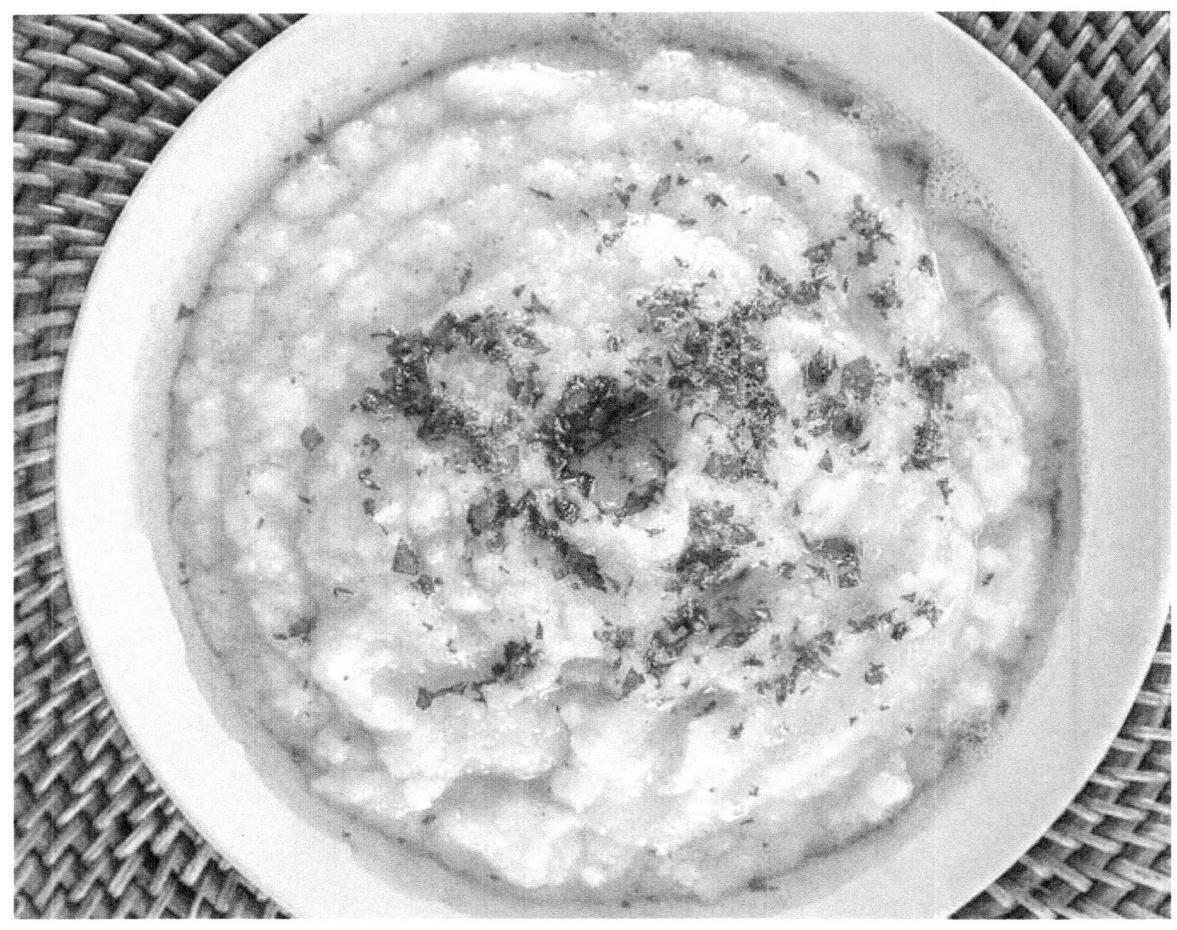

Celery root can be a taste that most people will not like. However, it's become a nice flavor when combined with other **Ingredients**.

Ingredients

- 1/4-pound parsnip~ peeled and sliced into 1" thick slices
- 1/2-pound celery root peeled and cubed into 1-1/2" chunks
- 1 cup nonfat milk, room temperature
- 1/8 cup green onion for garnish
- 1 Tablespoon butter, room temperature
- 1/4-pound turnips, peeled and cut into 1/2" cubes
- 1 teaspoon kosher salt
- 3/4 teaspoon coarse ground pepper

Directions

In a large stew pot add the parsnips, celery root, and turnips then add water to cover vegetables.

Once stew pot is boiling drop heat to a simmer and cook for 20 minutes.

Drain the vegetables and allow to cool for 6 minutes.

In a blender add milk, butter, pepper, salt, and vegetables, blend on puree until creamlike.

Pour puree into a serving dish, add the green onion, and then serve.

TIP:

If need to put the only half of the vegetables and other **Ingredients** into the blend at a time. Until all the **Ingredients** have been blended.

First Baby Peas

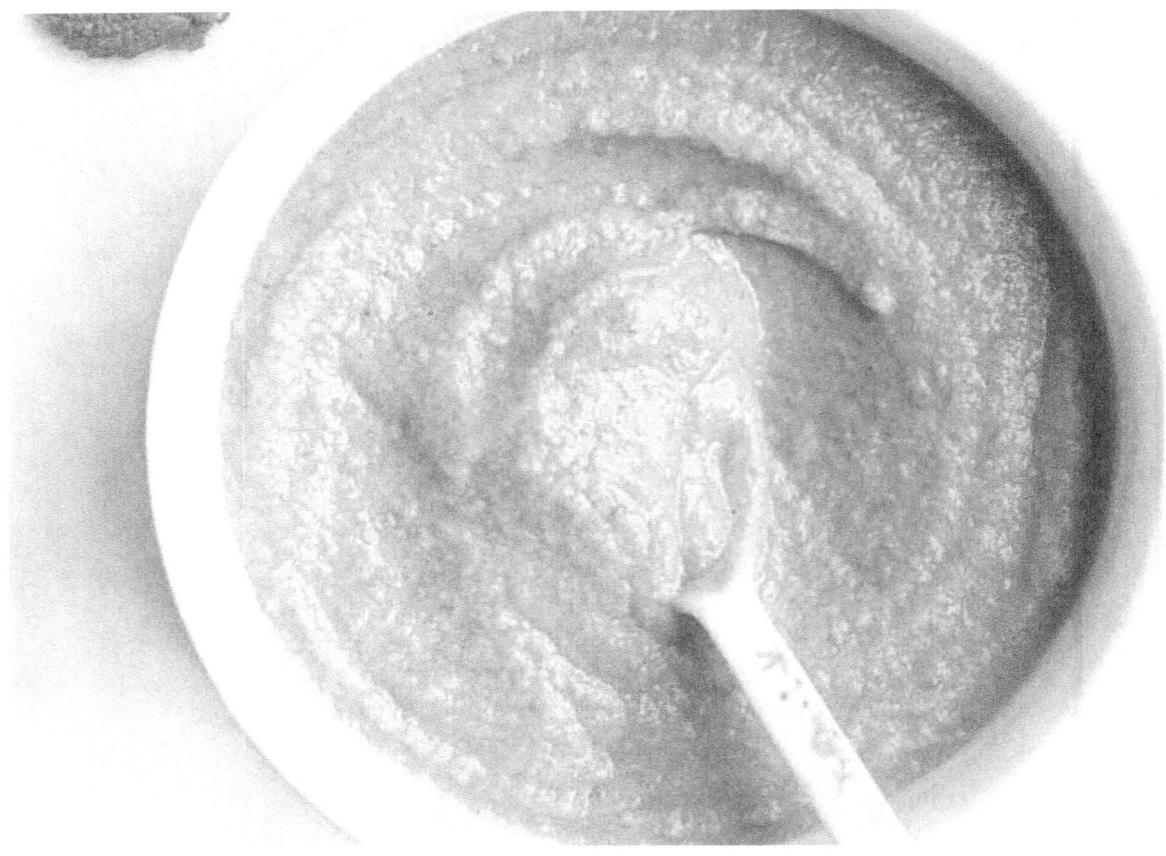

I know most babies don't like peas. However, this recipe is made with your own breast milk. This means more than like likely, your baby will eat this puree.

Ingredients

- 3 cups fresh peas
- 1/2 cup breast milk, fresh or frozen

Directions

Set a steamer basket into a pot and fill with water. Water should be right under stream but not overflowing into the basket.

Bring the water to a rapid boil.

Then, add the peas, and cover.

Steam for 20 minutes then removes from the pot.

Add the milk and peas into a blender and blend on high for 1 minute.

Serve

TIP:

I know this is a lot of food for a baby. Don't worry, you can pour the puree into an ice cube tray. All you need to do is allow the puree to cool then freeze them. Place into a freezer bag and heat when need. If you use a microwave to heat the cubes make sure not to heat for more than 30 seconds.

Papaya

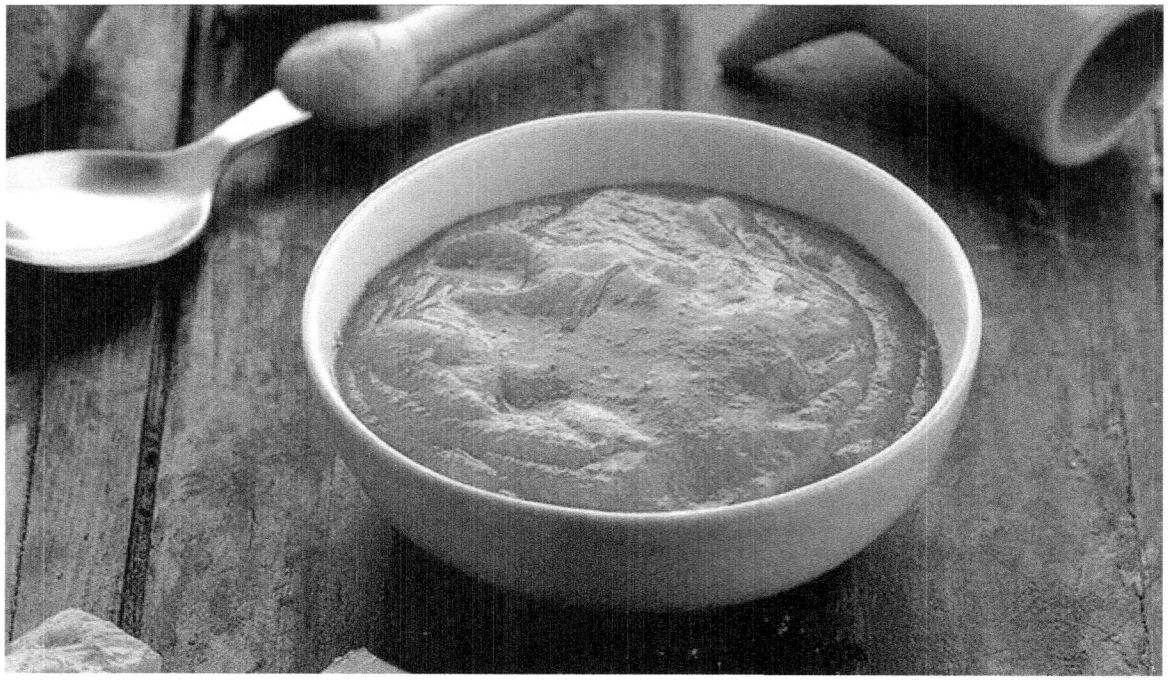

Simple tasty Papaya puree for a baby.

Ingredients

- 1/2 cup chopped Papaya
- Water - as needed

Directions

Clean the papaya under running tap water.

Peel the skin off using a vegetable peeler.

Cut into half and scoop out the seeds with a spoon.

Cut the fruit into small cubes.

Place into a blender and blend on puree setting for 1 minute or until smooth. Add the water as needed.

Place into a bowl and serve.

TIP:

Any leftover can be stored in an airtight continue for 2 days.

Creamy Provencal Chicken

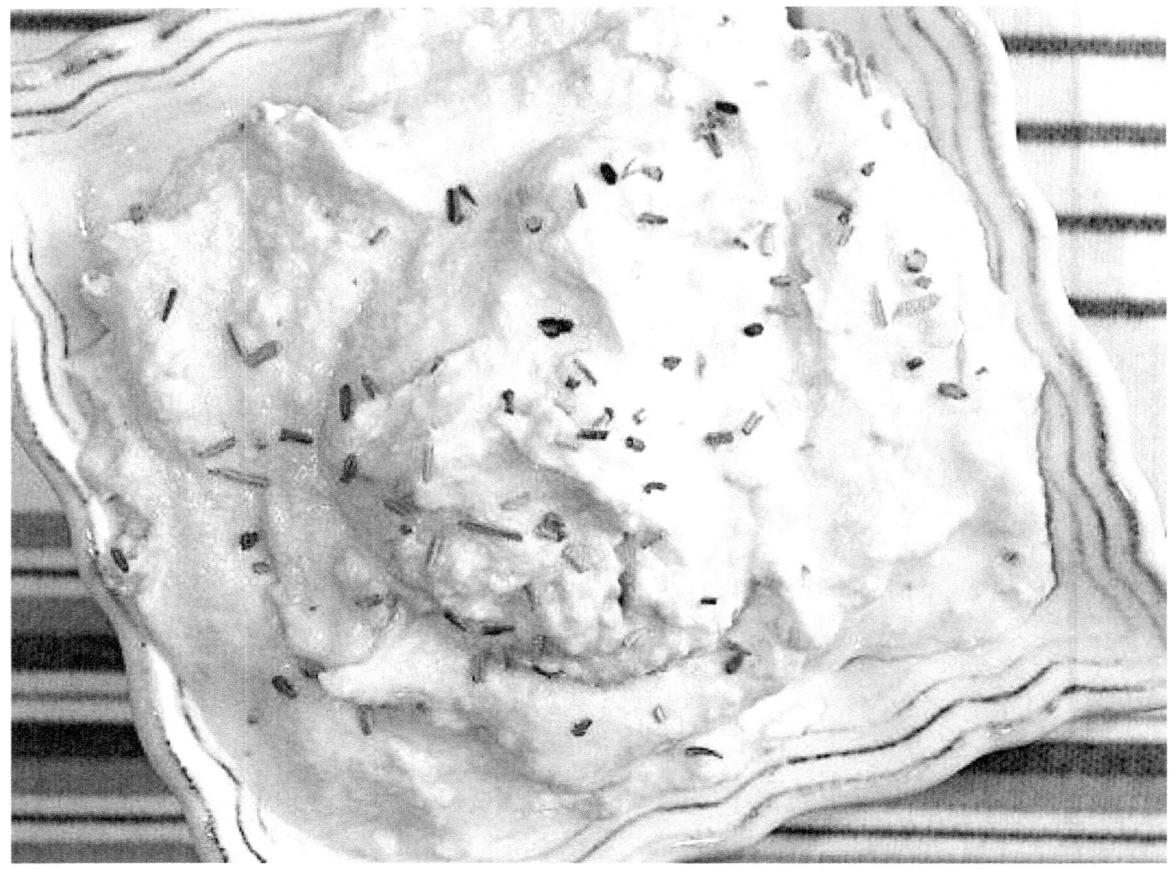

This combination of flavors is different, however, not too overwhelming, and with only a few **Ingredients**, you'll have a puree for the whole family.

Ingredients

- 1 organic chicken breast
- 1/4 cup low-sodium organic vegetable broth
- 1 tablespoon extra-virgin olive oil
- 2 tablespoons soft cheese
- 1/2 teaspoon marjoram

Directions

Cut the chicken breast into 1/2-inch-thick pieces.

Place a medium-size frying pan, over medium-high heat and add the olive oil 1 minute.

Place the marjoram and chicken into the frying pan.

Cook for 5 minutes on each side until light brown.

Remove the chicken from the pan and place onto a plate to cool.

Place the chicken into a blender add cheese and broth.

Pulse for 2 minutes or until smooth can creamy.

Serve with rice

TIP:

Add the broth a little at a time. Remember not to have a thin puree. The puree is to be thick.

Carrot, Mango, and Apple Puree

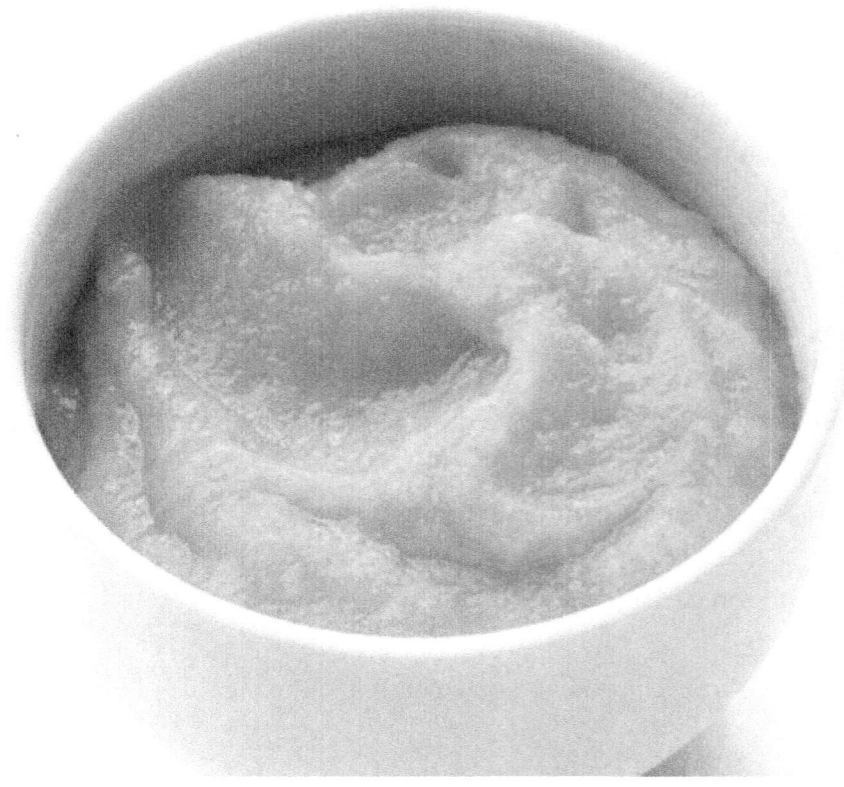

This recipe combines a vegetable with fruits. The kids would never know they are eating a vegetable.

Ingredients

- 3 large organic carrots
- 1 large organic mango
- 2 small organic Granny Smith apples

Directions

Preheat the oven to 350f

Line a cookie sheet with a parchment paper and place to the side

Using vegetable peeler peel the carrots and place into a bowl.

Peel the mango then cut into chunks.

Cut the apples into halves and remove the seeds.

Place the cut vegetables and fruits onto the cookie sheet and place into the oven.

Cook for 25 minutes then remove the cookie sheet and allow to cool 10 minutes.

Place the cooked vegetables and fruits into a food processor and pulse until creamy.

Pour into an airtight container and place into the refrigerator.

Once chilled serve and enjoy

Chayote

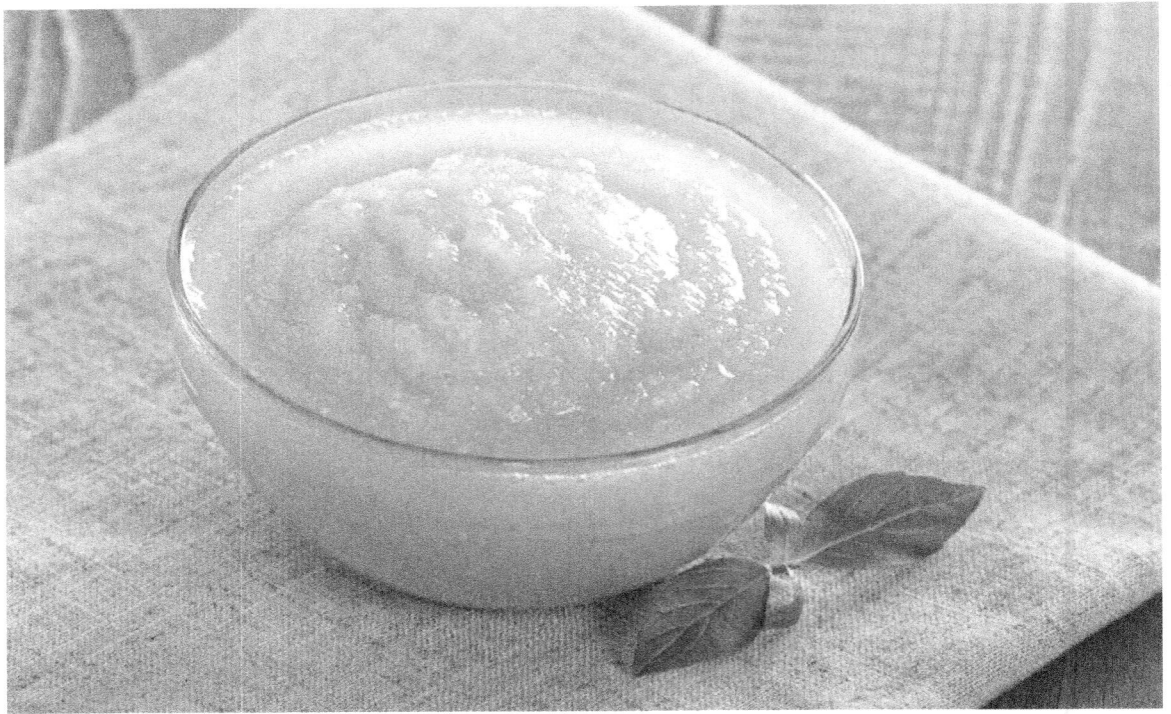

Chayote puree is something you can give to your baby. The taste is delicious and is light on the tummy.

Ingredients

- 1 piece of chayote squash
- 3 tablespoons water

Directions

Clean and remove the peel using a sharp knife.

Cut into half and remove the hard seed.

Cut each half into bite-size pieces.

Now, place the pieces into a pot and add water and steam until tender. About 10 minutes.

Remove the pieces from the water and pour into the blender.

Blend until smooth and creamy. Serve.

TIP:

Use bottled or boiled water when making this dish for your baby. Also, eat puree within 24 hours of making.

Cream of Mushroom Puree

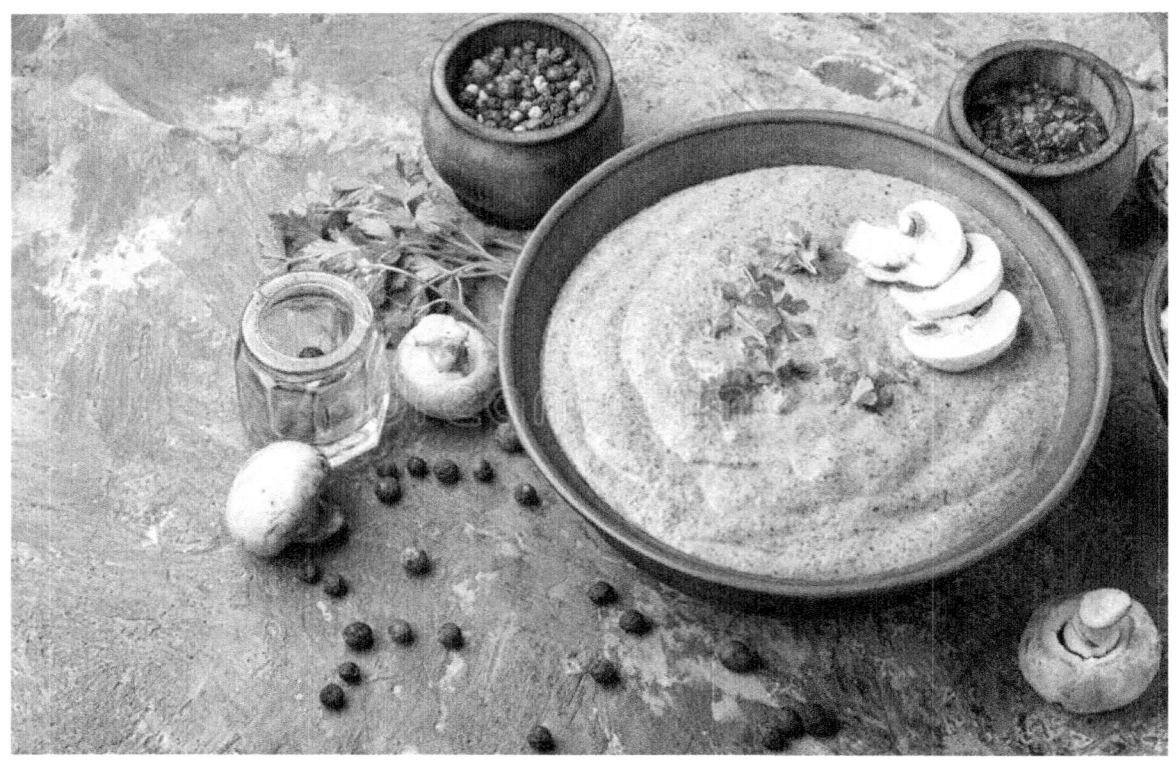

This is a really good recipe for mushroom lovers. You can eat this by itself or serve as an appetizer.

Ingredients

- 1/4 cup mushrooms (your choice)
- 3/4 cup heavy whipping cream
- 7/8 cup of butter
- 1/3 tablespoon Dijon mustard
- 1/3 teaspoon garlic powder
- 1/3 teaspoon paprika powder
- 2/3 teaspoon dried chives
- 2/3 teaspoon onion powder
- Salt and pepper to taste

Directions

Chop the mushrooms finely.

In a large frying pan over high heat add the butter and brown it.

Add the chopped mushrooms to the butter and cook until lightly golden.

Place the cream, mustard, salt, pepper, and seasonings, stir to mix well.

Drop the heat to low and cook for 15 minutes stirring often.

Remove the frying pan from the heat and cool for 5 minutes.

Puree using a hand mixer in a deep bowl, mix until smooth and a little thick.

Beef Stew for Babies

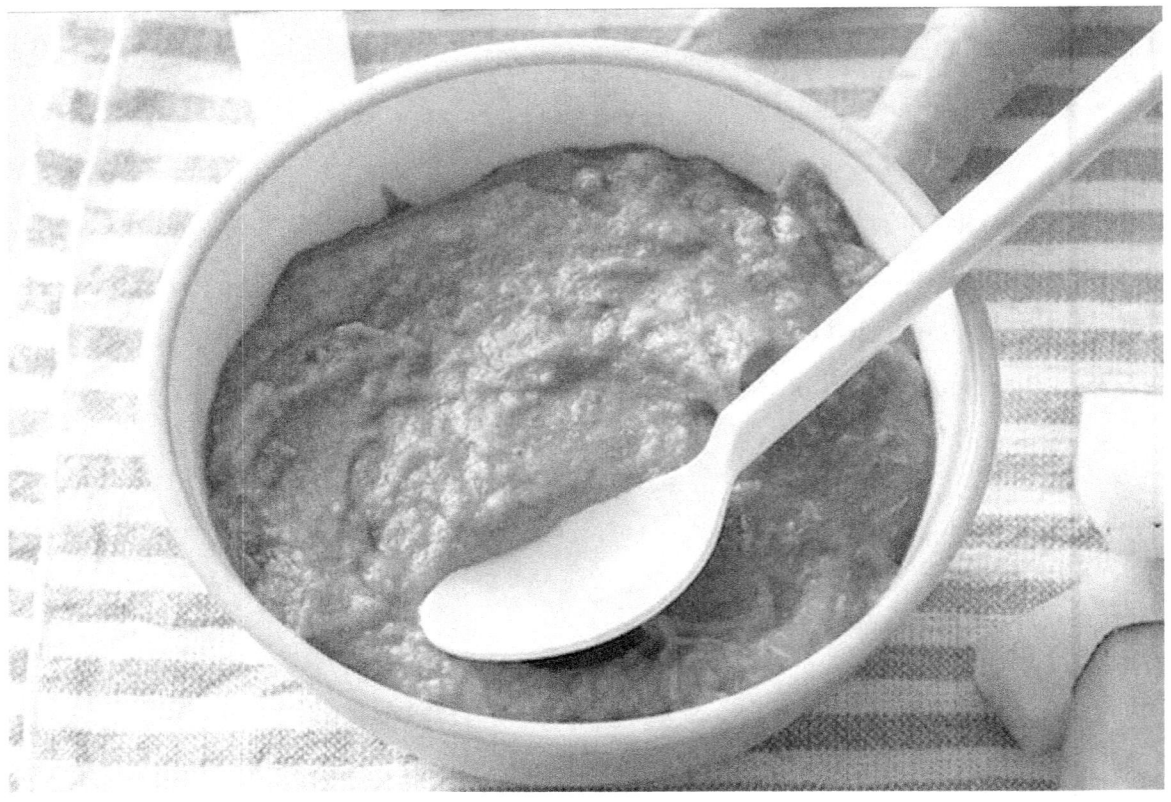

There is nothing better than a big bowl of beef stew on a cold winter's day. Loaded with beef, veggies, and flavor, this will soon be a go-to puree for a winter meal.

Ingredients

- 1/2 pound of boneless beef chuck roast, cut into 1/2-inch cubes
- 10 Baby Carrots, peeled and chopped
- 1 Medium Potato, peeled, cut into 1-inch cubes
- 2 Teaspoons olive oil
- 1/4 small onion, chopped
- ⅟ Cup water

Directions

In a heavy bottom pan, heat the oil over medium-high heat.

Once hot add the beef brown for 3 minutes on each side.

Add in the carrots, potatoes, onion, and water

Stir to combine the in **Ingredients**

Bring to a boil and then reduce to a low heat setting.

Cover with a lid that fits pot and cook for 1 hour and 30 minutes.

Allow to cool for about 10-12 minutes before pouring into a food processor.

Puree on high for a minute or until smooth.

Serve in bowls with toasted bread.

Sugar- free Fig Puree

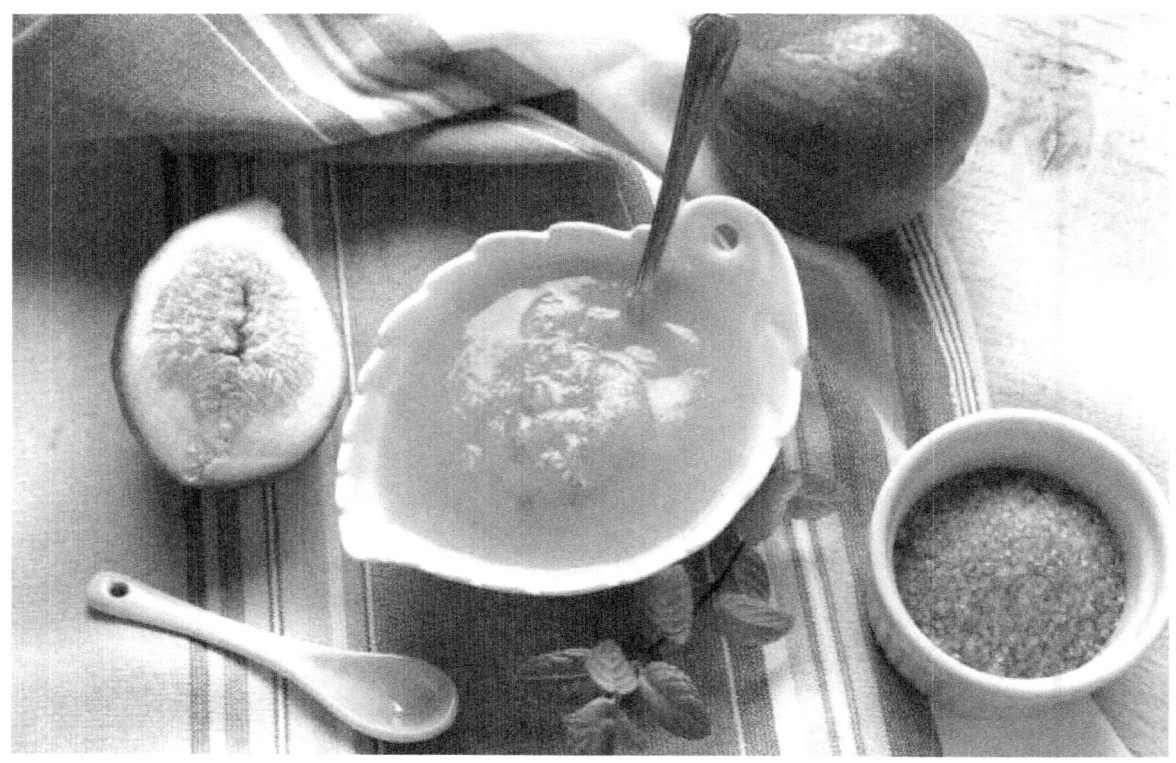

We all are looking for something sweet to eat. However, we don't want the added sugar. That's where this fig puree comes in handy. Not only is it gluten free, nut free, dairy free, egg free, it's sugar-free.

Ingredients

- 8 large fresh organic fig

Directions

Wash and remove the stems from the figs.

Cut each fig into fours and place into a blender.

Blend on puree setting until smooth.

Potato Puree with Garlic

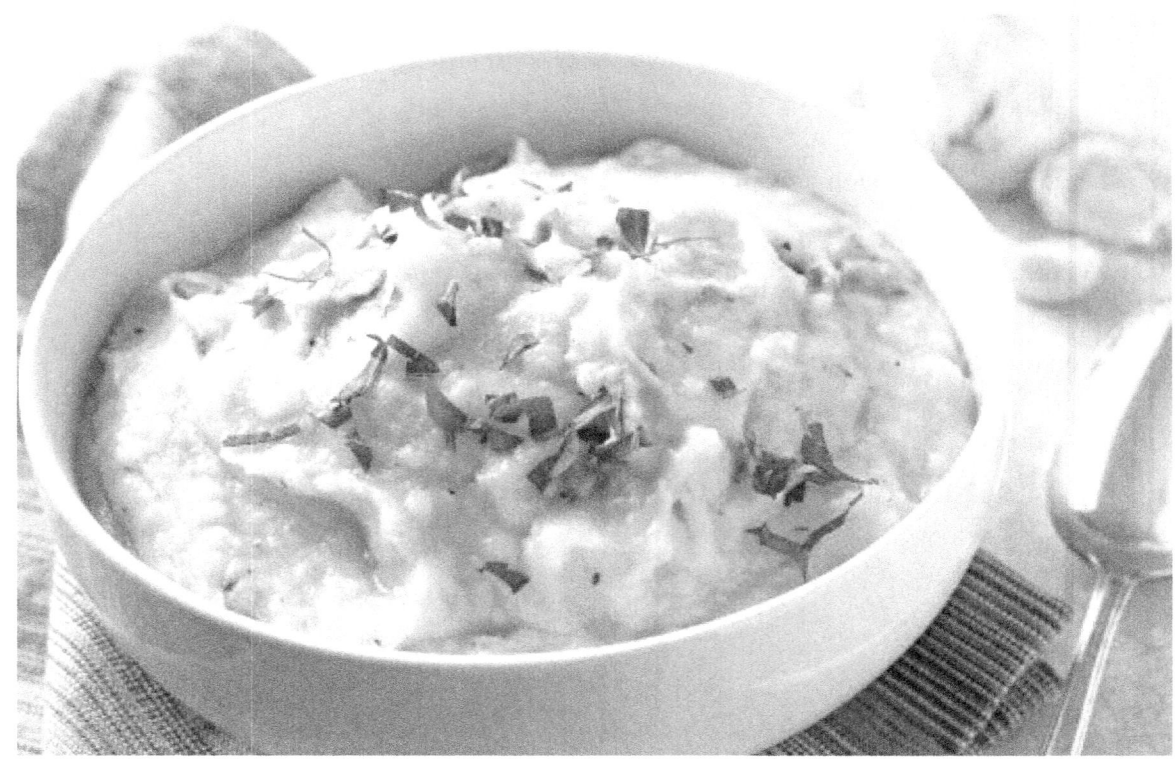

These mashed potatoes have garlic and butter flavor that everyone will enjoy

Ingredients

- 1-pound potatoes
- 1/4 cup heavy cream
- 4 tablespoons unsalted butter
- 2 garlic cloves
- Salt and freshly ground pepper to taste

Directions

Peel the potatoes and cut into 2-inch chunks

In a medium stew pan, cover potatoes and garlic with cold water.

Bring the water to a boil and cook over high heat 15 minutes.

Remove the potatoes and garlic and place into a medium-size bowl.

Put in the butter and cream then mix with a hand mixer until smooth.

Add the salt and pepper, stir to mix well and serve hot.

Lamb Puree

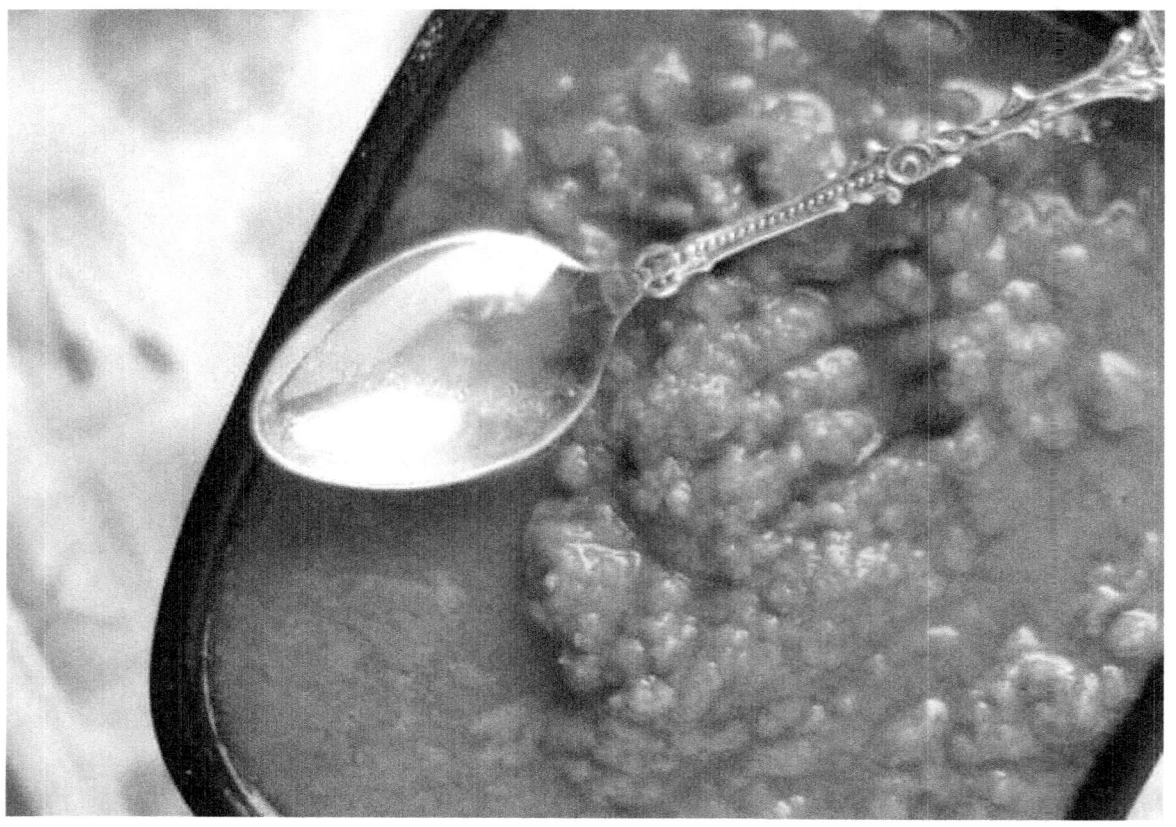

I have noticed that my kids will eat lamb this way. However, they want to eat it in lamb steaks.

Ingredients

- 1 teaspoon Olive oil
- 1 small lamb fillet
- 1 small potato
- 1 small carrot

Directions

In a hot pan add the olive oil and the lamb fillet.

Cook fillet until well done.

Remove from pan and place on a paper towel to drain.

Place the potato and carrot into a steamer, cook until soft

Place meat and vegetables in a blender and blend for 1 minute on puree or until smooth.

TIP:

Leftovers and be stored in the freezer for no more than 3 months.

Really Easy Apple Puree

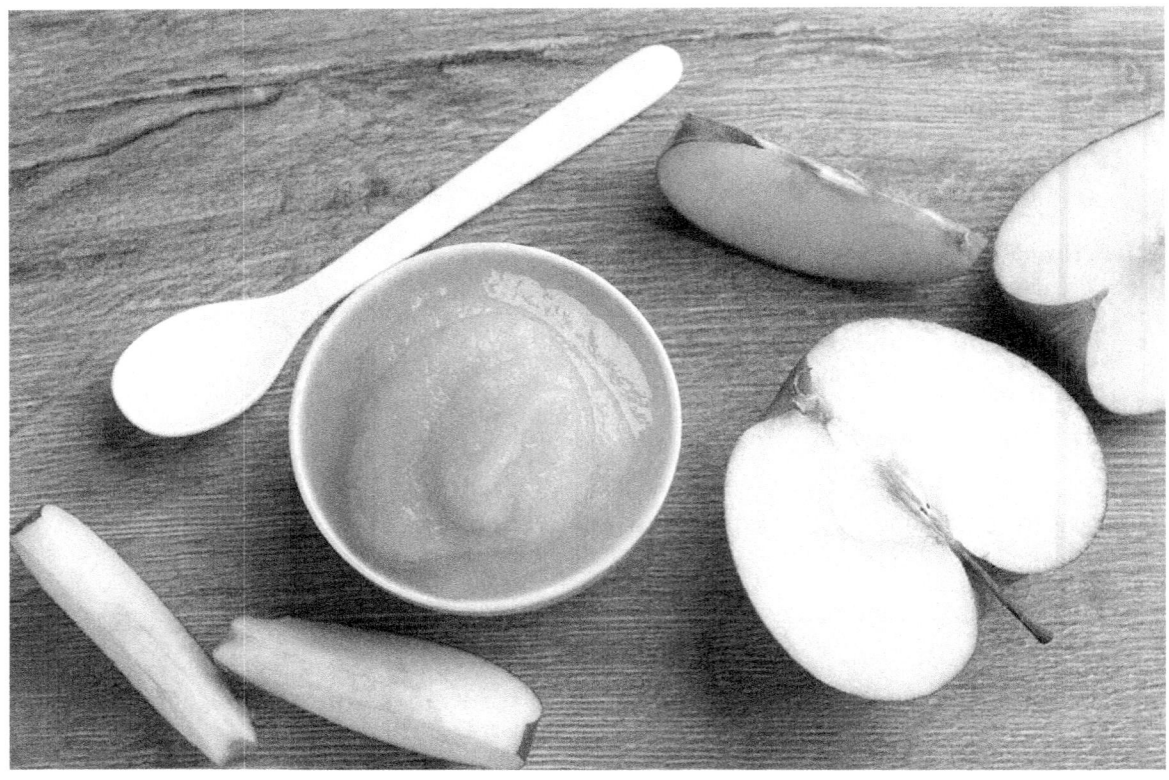

This recipe is a quick, simple, and healthy apple puree.

Ingredients

- 5 medium-sized red and green organic apples
- 1 teaspoon ground cinnamon
- 1 tablespoon low-calorie sweetener

Directions

Wipe the apples off then remove the peel, cut into halves and remove seeds.

In a large pan add the apples and cover with water.

Bring the water and apples to a rapid boil then lower heat to a simmer. Cook until tender.

Drain the water from the apples.

Place apples into a blender and the cinnamon and sweetener.

Blend until smooth.

Pour into a bowl and place in the

Fridge to cool for 30 minutes.

Watermelon

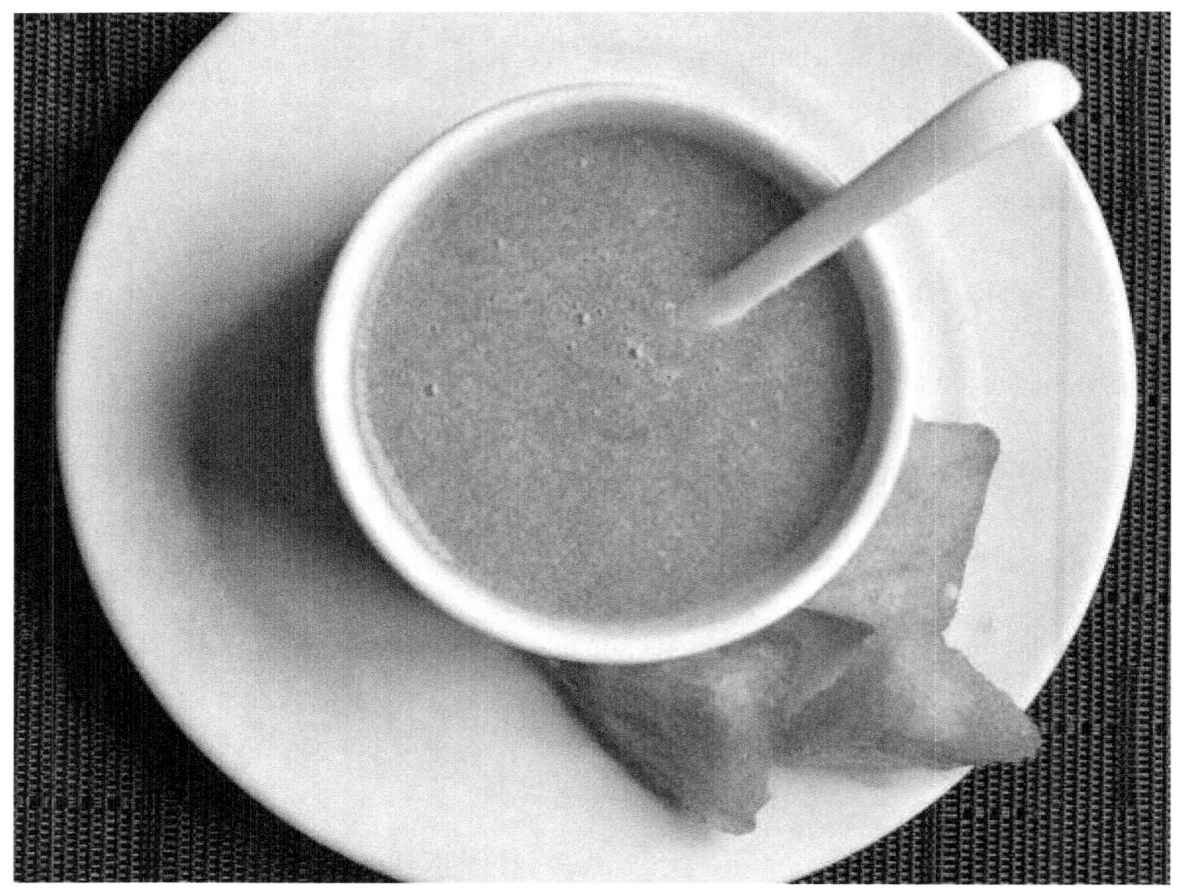

This juice from a fresh watermelon is combined with some fresh mint leaves to make this puree.

Ingredients

- 1 cup fresh watermelon
- 2-tablespoons water
- 1 tablespoon fresh mint leaves, chopped

Directions

Remove the seeds and cut watermelon meat from the rind.

Cut the watermelon into cubes. You only need a cup of the watermelon.

In a blender add the water and watermelon cubes.

Blend on puree setting until smooth.

Pour into a bowl and add the mint leaves.

Serve.

Zucchini Baby Food Puree

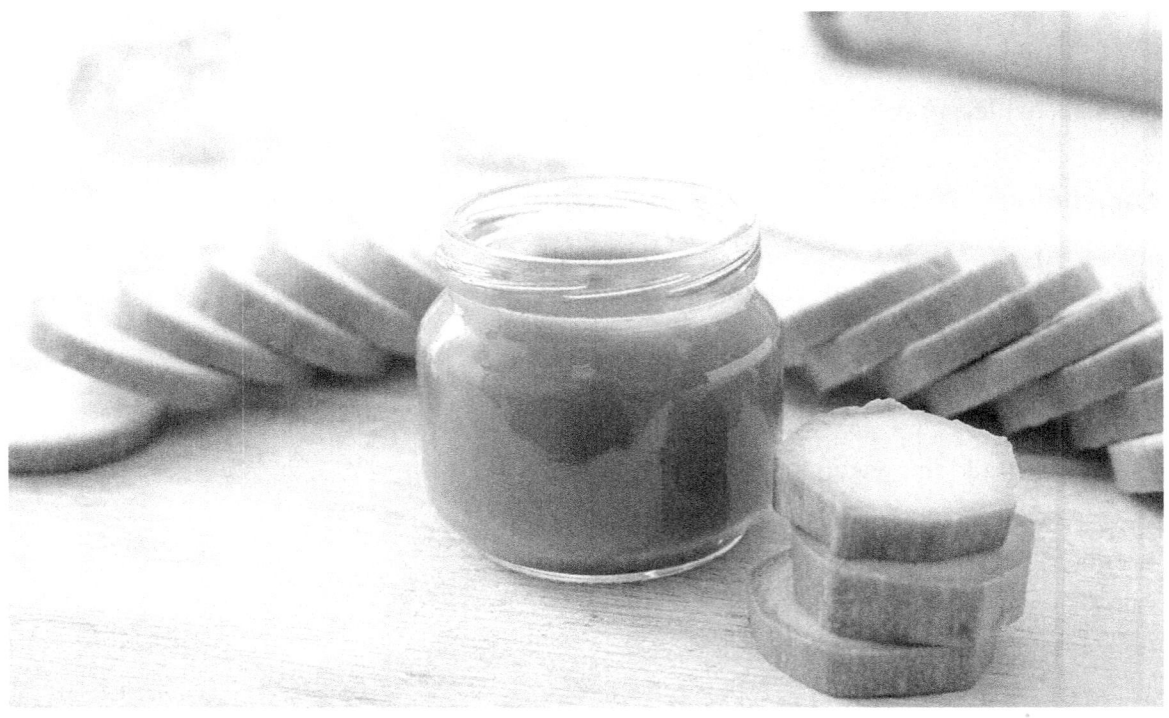

Zucchini makes a great puree for a baby and everyone.

Ingredients

- 2 small zucchinis, cut into 1-inch round slices
- 2 cups of water
- Salt to taste

Directions

Add 2 cups of water to boil in a saucepan.

Add the zucchini and lower heat to low, place a lid onto pot and cook for 8 minutes or until tender

Pour zucchini into a food processor and puree until creamy.

Serve.

TIP:

Place leftovers in an airtight container and store in the refrigerator for no more than 3 days. You can double the recipe and store in the freezer no more than 3 months.

White Bean Puree

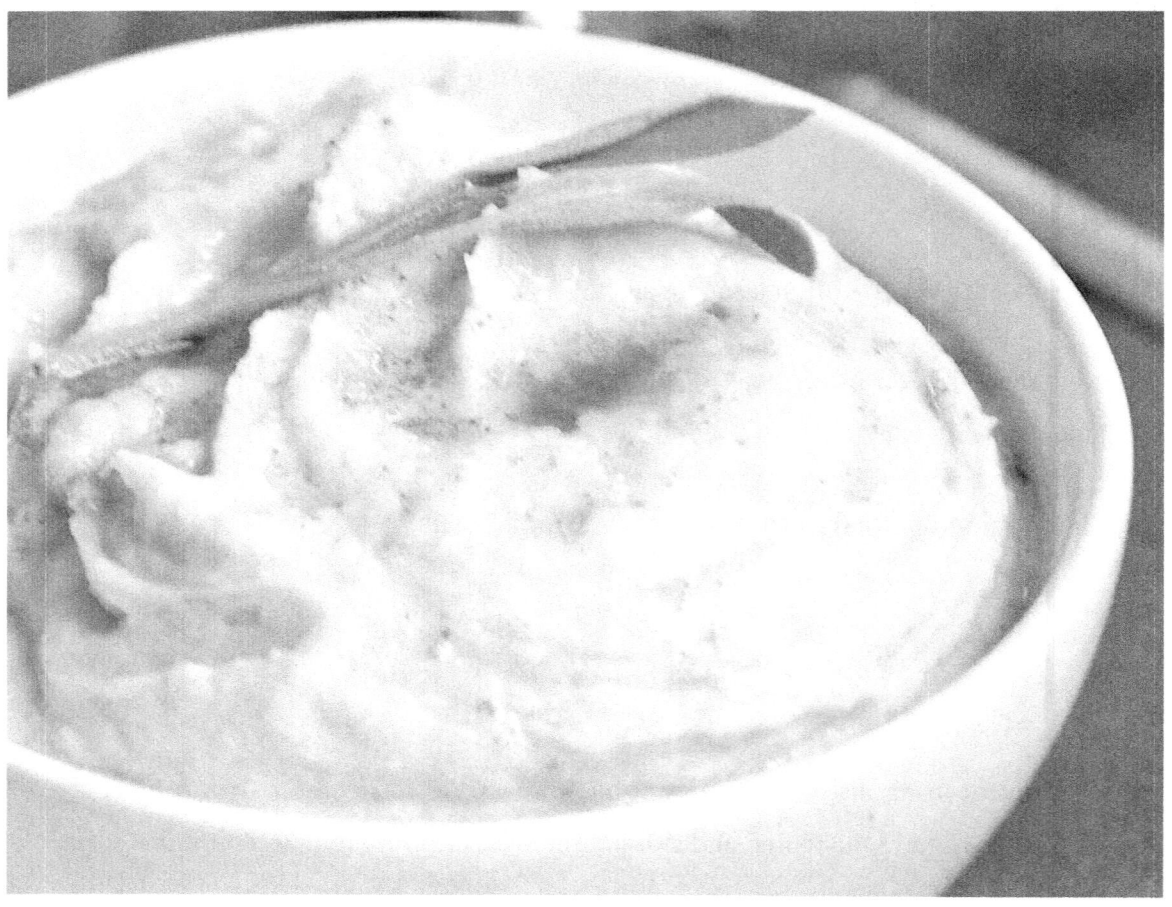

White beans and cornbread make a good meal. However, if you have a small child, they may not be able to eat beans whole. That's where this puree comes in handy.

Ingredients

- 2- Cans white beans 15-ounce, drained and rinsed
- 1 cup low-sodium chicken broth
- 1 small onion, diced
- 1 garlic clove, chopped
- 1 thyme sprig, chopped
- 3 tablespoons unsalted butter
- Salt and freshly ground pepper, to taste

Directions

Melt the butter in a medium saucepan, and add the garlic, onion, and thyme sprig medium-high heat for 10 minutes.

Pour half of the broth and 1 can of beans into the blender and blend until smooth.

Pour into a bowl.

Now add the onion mixture, the other can of beans and the last of broth into the blender and blend until smooth.

Pour mixture into the bowl and stir to combine. Add, the salt and pepper and stir once more.

Peach Puree

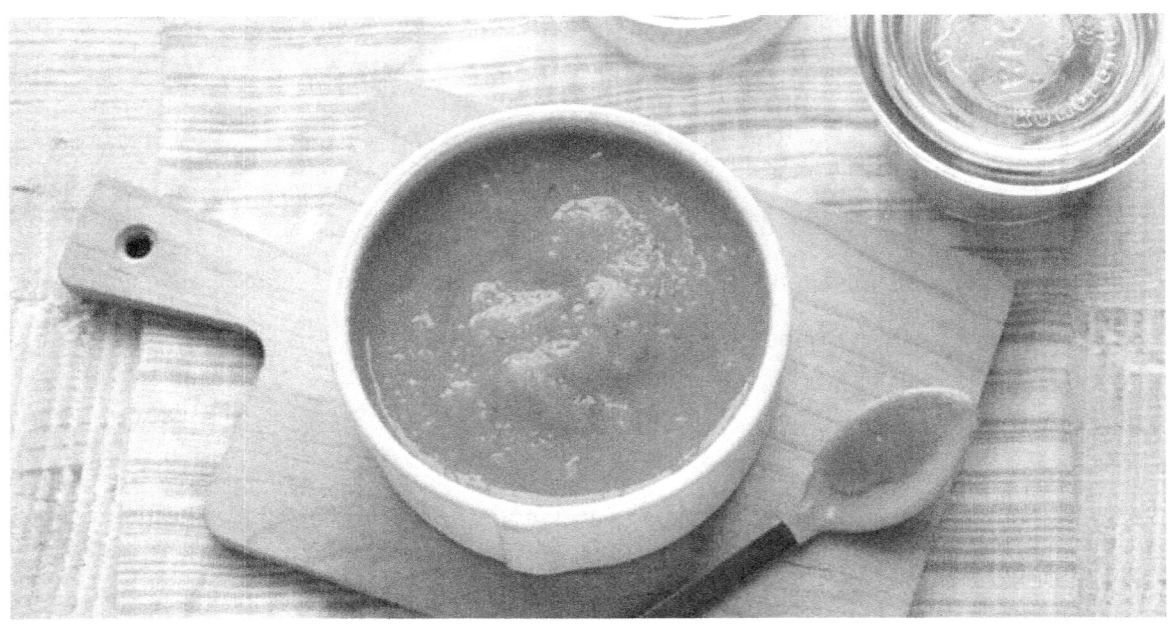

Peach puree with whipped topping is a true summertime treat. It's refreshing, creamy, and awesome.

Ingredients

- 2 cups fresh peaches
- 1/4 cup of water

Instruction

Wash peaches and cut into twos.

Remove seeds and place into a food processor.

Add the water and puree for 2 minutes or until smooth and creamy.

Pour into bowls and serve.

TIP:

A great topping for this puree is Greek yogurt.

Tomato Puree Recipe

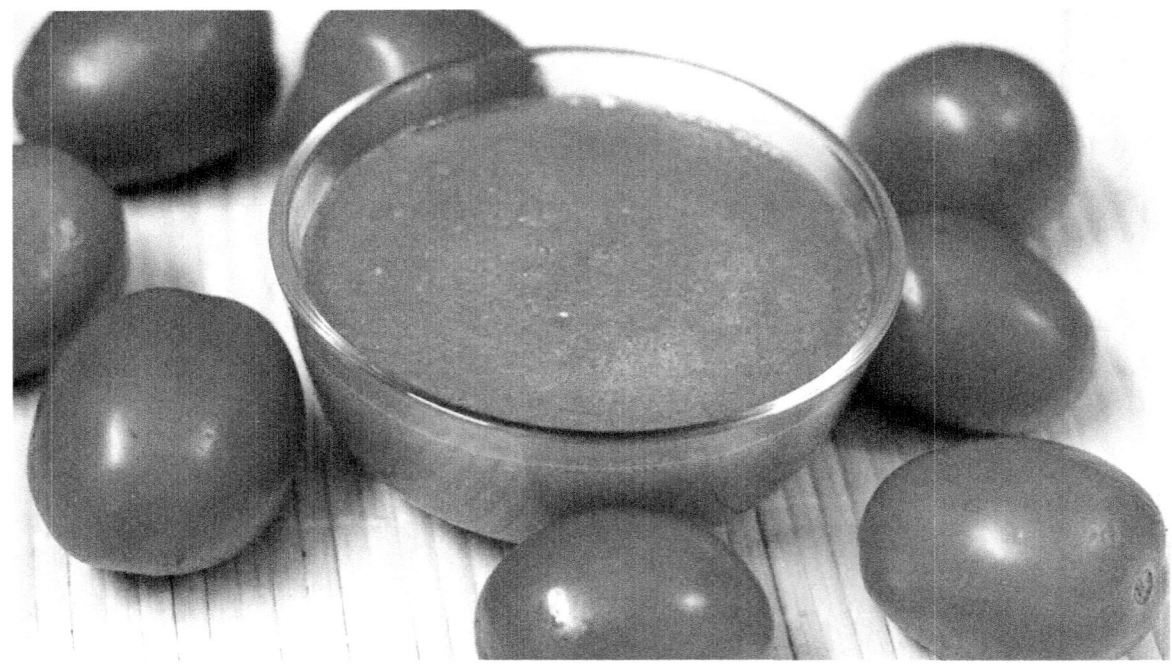

I like to make this puree and store it in the freezer until I need it. I make a great meal along with garlic, bread, or as a sauce for other dishes.

Ingredients

- 5 Red Plum Ripe Organic tomatoes
- 1/2 cup Water

Directions

Wash the tomatoes then cut 2 1/3-inch slices in the top of tomatoes.

Place into a sauce pot and cover with water.

Bring to a boil and cook for 4 minutes

Remove from heat and place tomatoes into a blender and blend for 1 minute or until smooth.

Pour into a serving bowl and serve.

TIP:

If you want to freeze the puree then pour evenly into freezer bags and store in the freezer. Keep in freeze up to 4 months.

Chicken, Rice, and Carrot

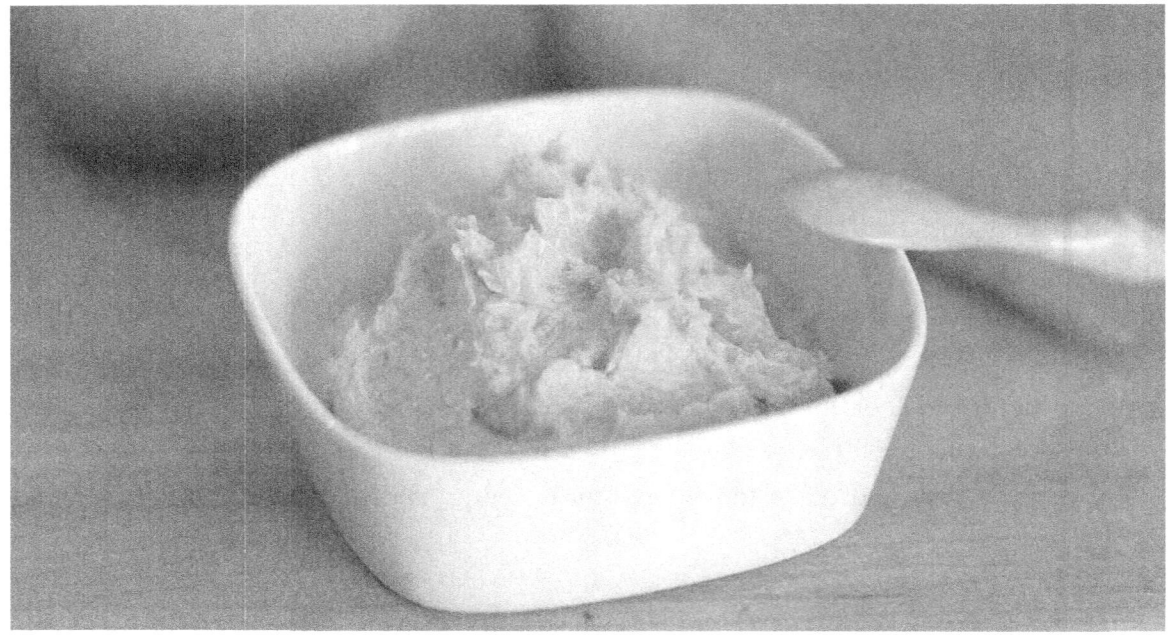

An entire meal in one serving. This recipe is great for a baby.

Ingredients

- 2 carrots, cut into pieces, peeled and steamed
- 3/4 cup chicken broth
- 1/2 cup pre-cooked chicken, cut into small cubes
- 1/3 Cup pre-cooked rice
- 1/4 cup applesauce
- 1 teaspoon rosemary

Directions

In a blender add the broth, chicken, carrots, applesauce, and rosemary.

Blend until smooth.

Serve.

Strawberry Puree

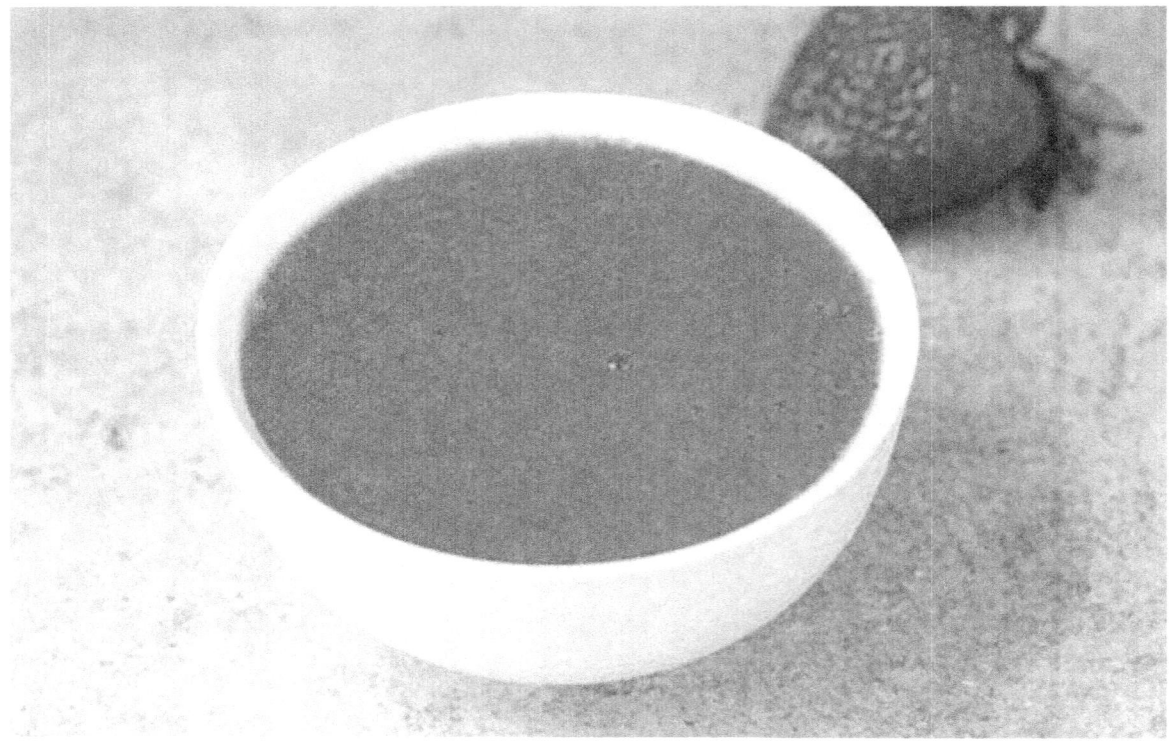

Strawberry Puree is something to have on hand for any occasion. You can add it to cakes, cookies, and more.

Ingredients

- 2 cups Strawberries

Directions

Wash strawberries and remove stems

Cut each one in half and then place it into a food processor.

Puree until thick.

Pour into a bowl and serve

TIP:

Place the puree into freezer bags and freeze up to 6 months.

Cooked Strawberry Puree

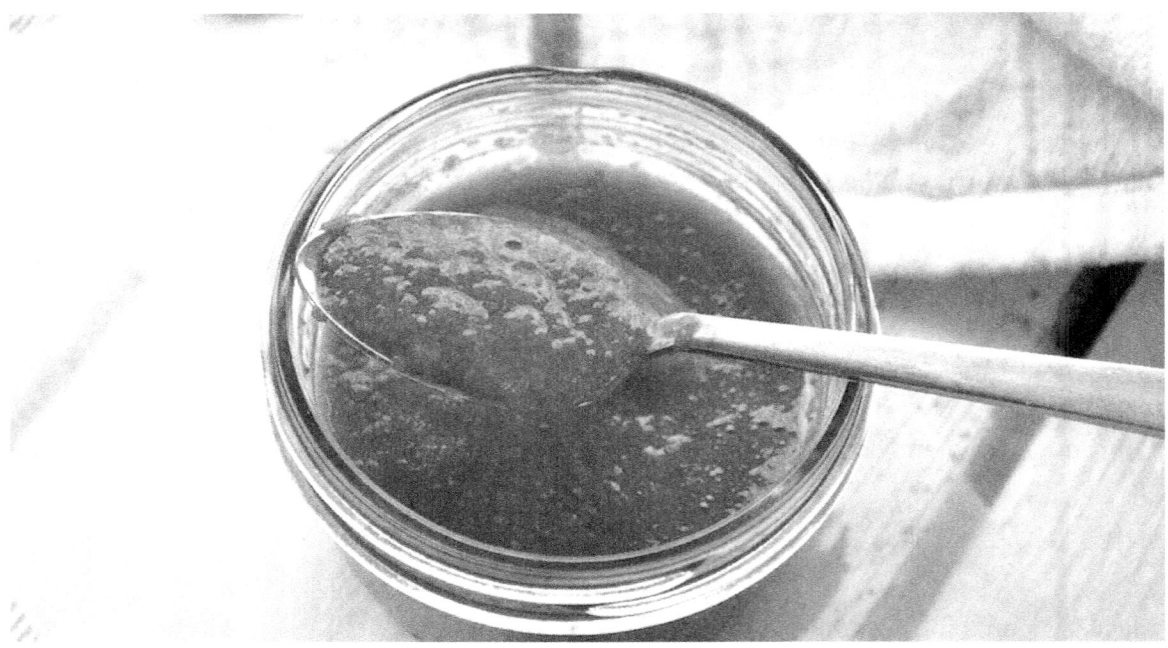

This recipe we use on pancakes and bread.

Ingredients

- 1/4 teaspoon white sugar
- 2 cups strawberries
- 1 tablespoon hot water

Directions

Wash and hull strawberries.

Cut into fours then place into a saucepan

In a cup add the sugar and water, stir until sugar has dissolved.

Pour sugar water into saucepan and place on medium, heat.

Once strawberries start to smell lower heat to a simmer for 10 minutes, stirring constantly.

Remove from heat and allow to cool 5 minutes.

Using a blender blend the strawberries on high until thick.

Place into a jar with a lid then store in the refrigerator for up to 1 month.

Cherry Puree

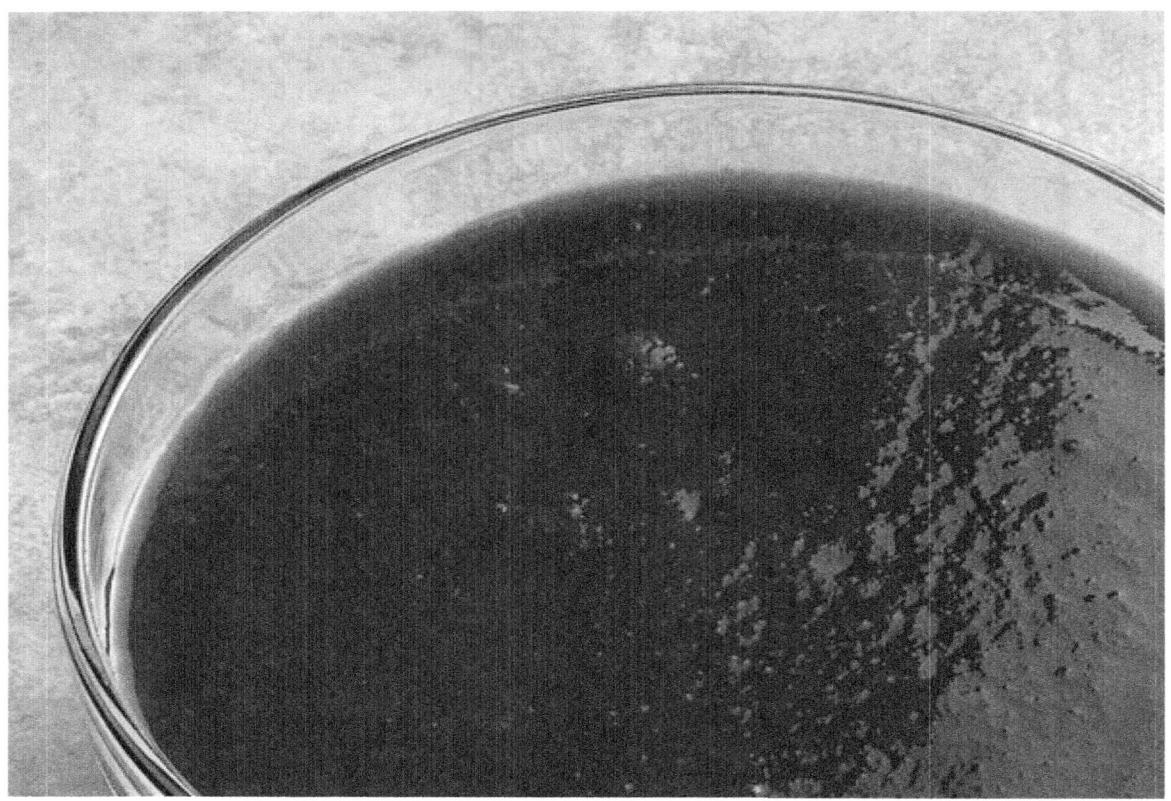

Cherries are a fruit that a lot of people look over. They thick all cherries are sour. However, that's not true. Cherries can be sour or sweet. This recipe will show the sweet side of this fruit.

Ingredients

- 1-pound fresh cherries
- 2 tablespoons freshly squeezed lemon juice
- 2 tablespoons granulated sugar,

Directions

Wash and remove the stem of the cherries.

Cut in half and remove the seeds.

Place cherries, sugar and lime juice into a food processor and puree until creamy and smooth.

Pour into a dish and serve.

TIP:

Add a little more sugar if needed. Place in the airtight container to store in the refrigerator for up to 3 days or freeze no more than 3 months.

Plum Puree

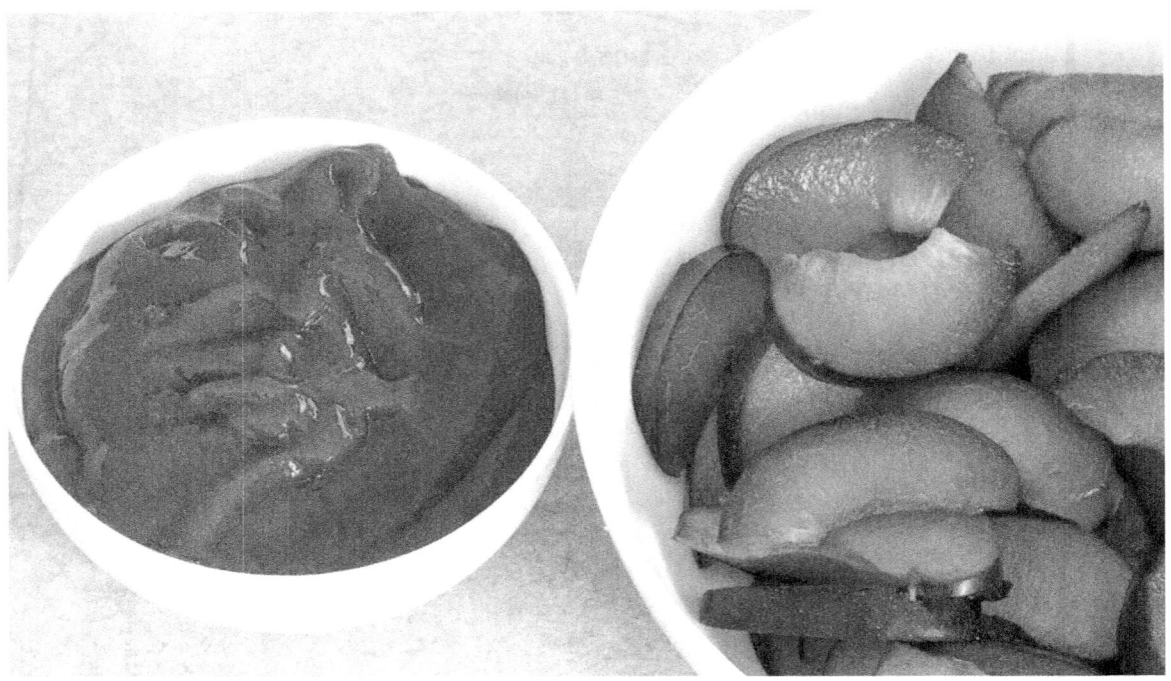

Toddler 1 year of age and older will enjoy this plum puree. You can add vanilla yogurt or apples for a nice surprise in taste.

Ingredients

- 4 small ripe plums

Directions

Wash then remove the pita from each plum.

In a pot and the plumps and water just to cover the plums.

Place pot on the stove over high heat.

Once plums start to boil reduce the heat to a simmer.

Place a lid on the pot and cook until soft.

Remove plums and cool 10 minutes.

Remove peel and place seemed plums into a blender.

Blend on puree setting for 2 minutes or until thick.

Remove from blender and pour into a bowl.

TIP:

Save some of the liquid from the pot. This you might need if the puree is too thick. Keep in mind to add only a teaspoon of liquid at a time until you like the consistency.

Conclusion

Please remember as you make these purees….

Combining food and liquid gradually into a blender or food processor will help keep the right texture for a puree. If you find the puree thin, then add food a little to make it thicken. If purees are too thick, you need to add liquid. The liquid can be water, broth, juice, or milk.

Best of luck to you as you make these awesome purees for your friends and family.

About the Author

Ivy's mission is to share her recipes with the world. Even though she is not a professional cook she has always had that flair toward cooking. Her hands create magic. She can make even the simplest recipe tastes superb. Everyone who has tried her food has astounding their compliments was what made her think about writing recipes.

She wanted everyone to have a taste of her creations aside from close family and friends. So, deciding to write recipes was her winning decision. She isn't interested in popularity, but how many people have her recipes reached and touched people. Each recipe in her cookbooks is special and has a special meaning in her life. This means that each recipe is created with attention and love. Every ingredient carefully picked, every combination tried and tested.

Her mission started on her birthday about 9 years ago, when her guests couldn't stop prizing the food on the table. The next thing she did was organizing an event where chefs from restaurants were tasting her recipes. This event gave her the courage to start spreading her recipes.

She has written many cookbooks and she is still working on more. There is no end in the art of cooking; all you need is inspiration, love, and dedication.

Author's Afterthoughts

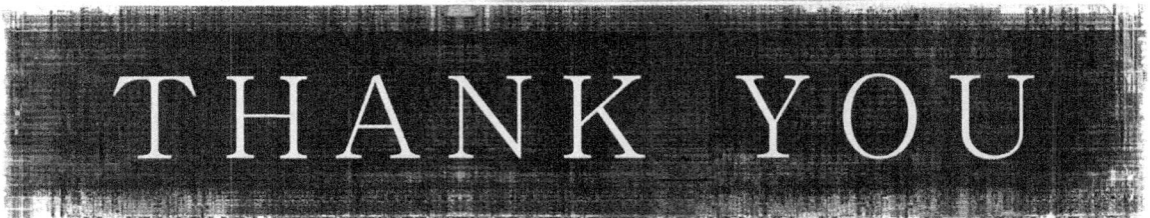

I am thankful for downloading this book and taking the time to read it. I know that you have learned a lot and you had a great time reading it. Writing books is the best way to share the skills I have with your and the best tips too.

I know that there are many books and choosing my book is amazing. I am thankful that you stopped and took time to decide. You made a great decision and I am sure that you enjoyed it.

I will be even happier if you provide honest feedback about my book. Feedbacks helped by growing and they still do. They help me to choose better content and new ideas. So, maybe your feedback can trigger an idea for my next book.

Thank you again

Sincerely

Ivy Hope

Printed in Great Britain
by Amazon